Transdermal
Delivery
of
Drugs

Volume I

Editors

Agis F. Kydonieus, Ph.D.
President
Hercon Laboratories Corporation
Subsidiary of Health-Chem Corporation
South Plainfield, New Jersey

Bret Berner, Ph.D.
Manager
Pharmaceutical Division
Ciba-Geigy Corporation
Ardsley, New York

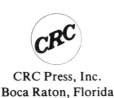

CRC Press, Inc.
Boca Raton, Florida

Library of Congress Cataloging-in-Publication Data

Transdermal delivery of drugs.

Includes bibliographies and index.
1. Ointments. 2. Skin absorption. 3. Drugs--
Controlled release. I. Kydonieus, Agis F., 1938-
II. Berner, Bret. [DNLM: 1. Administration, Topical.
2. Delayed-Action Preparations. 3. Drugs--administra-
tion & dosage. 4. Skin Absorption. WB 340 T7723]
RS201.03T7255 1987 615'.67 86-2585
ISBN 0-8493-6483-3 (set)
ISBN 0-8493-6484-1 (v. 1)
ISBN 0-8493-6485-X (v. 2)
ISBN 0-8493-6486-8 (v. 3)

Direct all inquiries to CRC Press, Inc., 2000 Corporate Blvd., N.W., Boca Raton, Florida, 33431.

International Standard Book Number 0-8493-6483-3 (set)
International Standard Book Number 0-8493-6484-1 (v. 1)
International Standard Book Number 0-8493-6485-X (v. 2)
International Standard Book Number 0-8493-6486-8 (v. 3)

Library of Congress Card Number 86-2585
Printed in the United States

PREFACE

The introduction of the first transdermal patch containing scopolamine brought about a tremendous interest in the usage of intact skin as a portal of entry of drugs into the systemic circulation of the body. Several transdermal products followed into the marketplace, in particular, devices containing nitroglycerin, clonidine, isosorbide dinitrate (Japan), and estradiol (Switzerland). Some two dozen drugs are now in different steps of transdermal product development. A plethora of transdermal development departments and companies have emerged. While the potential advantages of transdermal delivery such as (1) avoidance of hepatic "first-pass" metabolism, (2) maintenance of steady-state plasma levels of drug, and (3) convenience of dosing were readily identified, the limitations of the barrier and immune properties of skin are only now being defined. Continued technological advances are requiring either circumventing these responses of the skin or adroit identification of conditions in search of controlled-release therapies. The goals of these volumes are to collect the current knowledge to further research in transdermal delivery and to serve as an introduction to the novice.

The series of volumes is divided into four main sections pertaining to Methodology, The Transdermal Device, The Skin, and The Drug. For the recent practitioner in the field, an overview section has been included to provide a background about the controlled release devices, the diffusion of drugs through polymers, and the anatomy and biochemistry of skin.

In the methodology section, the techniques used to determine in vitro and in vivo skin permeation are presented. The special considerations concerning animal and human experimentation are described including in vivo methodology, skin condition, and individual variations.

A section on transdermal devices concludes the first volume. Here we asked scientists from six companies to discuss briefly their transdermal technology and product development areas.

The volume on skin contains chapters on the parameters affecting skin penetration, including a chapter on aging, pharmacokinetics of transdermal delivery, models for predicting the permeability of drugs through skin from the physicochemical parameters of the drug, the correlations among human skin, reconstituted skin, artificial membranes, and the potential of increasing skin permeability by the use of chemical enhancers or vehicles. Finally, a chapter on the crucial area of cutaneous toxicology describes contact dermatitis and microorganism growth and infections.

In the third volume, the drug parameters important to transdermal delivery are discussed. The thermodynamics governing transdermal delivery and models and typical approaches for prodrugs are also presented. Finally, a literature review of the permeability of drugs through the skin is presented. This compilation of existing skin permeation data should serve as a useful reference tool.

Obviously, in this rapidly expanding field, several important omissions must have occurred despite our effort to include significant developments known by 1984, when most of the manuscripts were collected. Nevertheless, we hope this effort will prove to be of value to scientists and product development engineers seeking up-to-date information in this area.

We are indebted to the authors for their cooperation in adhering to manuscript specifications and to Mrs. Robin Tyminski for her efforts in typing and assisting in the editorial endeavors. Finally, we would like to thank the management of Health-Chem Corporation, the parent of Hercon Laboratories, who have been strong advocates of controlled release for many years and have given the editors all the support required to complete this undertaking.

Agis F. Kydonieus
Bret Berner

THE EDITORS

Agis F. Kydonieus, Ph.D., is President of Hercon Laboratories Corporation, a subsidiary of Health-Chem Corporation, New York. Dr. Kydonieus graduated from the University of Florida in 1959 with a B.S. degree in Chemical Engineering (summa cum laude) and received his Ph.D. from the same school in 1964.

Dr. Kydonieus is a founder of the Controlled Release Society and has served as a member of the Board of Governors, Program Chairman, Vice President, and President. He is presently a trustee of the Society. He is also founder of Krikos, an international Hellenic association of scientists, and has served a treasurer and a member of its Board of Directors. He is also a member of the editorial board of the *Journal of Controlled Release,* and a member of many societies including the American Association of Pharmaceutical Scientists, American Institute of Chemical Engineers, and the Society of Plastics Engineers.

Dr. Kydonieus is the author of over 125 patents, publications, and presentations in the field of controlled release and biomedical devices. He is the Editor of *Controlled Release Technologies* and *Insect Suppression with Controlled Release Pheromone Systems,* both published with CRC Press.

Bret Berner, Ph.D., is Manager of Basic Pharmaceutics Research for CIBA-GEIGY, Inc. Dr. Berner received his B.A. degree from the University of Rochester in 1973 and his Ph.D. from the University of California at Los Angeles in 1978. Before joining CIBA-GEIGY in 1985, he was Director of Research, Hercon Division of Health-Chem Corporation. Dr. Berner also held the position of staff scientist with Proctor & Gamble, Co. following his graduation from UCLA.

Dr. Berner's current research directs novel drug delivery research groups including transdermal, gastrointestinal, and other delivery routes, polymer systems, pharmacokinetics, pharmacodynamics, and analytical chemistry.

CONTRIBUTORS

Bret Berner, Ph.D.
Manager
Pharmaceuticals Division
Ciba-Geigy Corporation
Ardsley, New York

Donald Bissett, Ph.D.
Proctor & Gamble Company
Miami Valley Laboratories
Cincinnati, Ohio

Yie W. Chien, Ph.D.
Professor and Chairman
Department of Pharmaceutics
Rutgers University
Piscataway, New Jersey

Gary W. Cleary, Ph.D.
President
Cygnus Research Corporation
San Mateo, California

Gordon L. Flynn, Ph.D.
Professor of Pharmaceutics
College of Pharmacy
University of Michigan
Ann Arbor, Michigan

Robert M. Gales, M.S.
Senior Product Development Manager
Product Development Area
Alza Corporation
Palo Alto, California

Timothy A. Hagen
College of Pharmacy
University of Michigan
Ann Arbor, Michigan

Dean S.T. Hsieh, Ph.D.
President
Conrex Pharmaceutical Corporation
Edison, New Jersey

Allan Hymes, Ph.D.
Medical Consultant
LecTec Corporation
Minneapolis, Minnesota

Aziz Karim, Ph.D.
Director
Department of Pharmacokinetics
G.D. Searle & Company
Skokie, Illinois

Alec D. Keith, Ph.D.
Professor
Department of Biophysics
Pennsylvania State Univeristy
University Park, Pennsylvania

Agis F. Kydonieus, Ph.D.
President
Hercon Laboratories Corporation
Subsidiary of Health-Chem
  Corporation
New York, New York

Howard Maibach, M.D.
Professor
Department of Dermatology
University of California
  at San Francisco
San Francisco, California

Arthur S. Obermayer, Ph.D.
Chairman of the Board
Moleculon, Inc.
Cambridge, Massachusetts

Nikolaos A. Peppas, Sc.D.
Professor
School of Chemical Engineering
Purdue University
West Lafayette, Indiana

Marilou Powers Cramer, B.S.
Director of Clinical Sciences
Alza Corporation
Palo Alto, California

David Rolf, Ph.D.
Director of Medical Services
LecTec Corporation
Minneapolis, Minnesota

Jane E. Shaw, Ph.D.
President
Alza Corporation
Palo Alto, California

Ward M. Smith
College of Pharmacy
University of Michigan
Ann Arbor, Michigan

Ronald C. Wester, Ph.D.
Assistant Research Dermatologist
Department of Dermatology
University of California
 at San Francisco
San Francisco, California

TABLE OF CONTENTS

Volume I

Section I: Overview

Chapter 1

FUNDAMENTALS OF TRANSDERMAL DRUG DELIVERY

Agis F. Kydonieus

TABLE OF CONTENTS

I. INTRODUCTION

Controlled release may be defined as a technique or method in which active chemicals are made available to a specified target at a rate and duration designed to accomplish an intended effect. A definition perhaps more acceptable to the chemist and engineer may be the permeation-moderated transfer of an active material from a reservoir to a target surface to maintain a predetermined concentration or emission level for a specified period of time. Transdermal drug delivery can, therefore, be defined as the controlled release of drugs through intact skin.

In this book we will further limit the definition of transdermal systems to the newly introduced polymeric devices designed for prolonged delivery of drug through intact skin.

II. RATIONALE FOR TRANSDERMAL CONTROLLED RELEASE MEDICATION

During the last decade, controlled release technology has received increasing attention in the face of a growing awareness that substances ranging from drugs to agricultural chemicals are frequently excessively toxic and sometimes ineffective when administered or applied by conventional means. Thus, conventionally administered drugs in the form of pills, capsules, injectables, and ointments are introduced into the body as pulses that usually produce large fluctuations of drug concentrations in the bloodstream and tissues and consequently, unfavorable patterns of efficacy and toxicity.

The process of molecular diffusion through polymers and synthetic membranes has been used as an effective and reliable means of attaining transdermal controlled release of drugs and pharmacologically active agents. Central to the development of transdermal controlled delivery systems is the synthesis of the principles of molecular transport in polymeric materials and those of pharmacokinetics and pharmacodynamics. In transdermal drug delivery, pharmacokinetics is an important consideration because target tissues are seldom directly accessible, and drugs must be transported from the portal of entry on the body through a variety of biological interfaces to reach the desired receptor site. During this transport process, the drug can undergo severe biochemical degradation and, thereby, produce a delivery pattern at the receptor site that differs markedly from the pattern of drug release into the system.

A. Conventional Delivery vs. Transdermal Controlled Release of Medication

Conventionally, active agents are most often administered to a system by nonspecific, periodic applications. For example, in medical treatment, drugs are introduced at intervals by ingestion of pills or liquids or by injection. The drugs then circulate throughout much of the body, and the concentration of the active agent rises to high levels, system-wide, at least initially.[1] Both by injection and orally, the initially high concentrations may be toxic and cause side effects both to the target organ and neighboring structures. As time passes, the concentration diminishes, owing to natural metabolic processes, and a second dose must be administered to prevent the concentration from dropping below the minimum effective level. Such responses are shown in Figure 1. This situation is, of course, very inconvenient and difficult to monitor, and careful calculations of the amount of residual active agent must be made to avoid overdosing. The close attention required, together with the fact that large amounts of the drug are lost in the vicinity of the target organ, make this type of delivery inefficient and costly. In addition, side effects owing to drugs misdirected to nontarget tissues are also possible.

Cowsar has discussed a hypothetical drug that is effective at 5 ± 2 mg/kg (below 3 mg/kg ineffective, above 7 mg/kg toxic) and has a half-life in vivo of 8 hr; his regimen calls

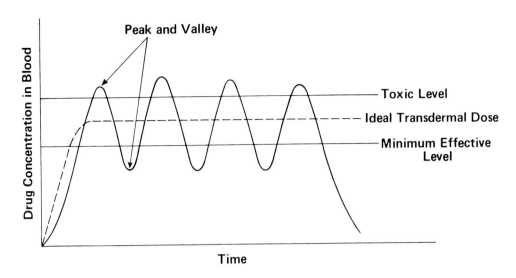

FIGURE 1. Hypothetical blood level pattern from a conventional multiple dosing schedule, and the idealized pattern from a transdermal controlled release system.

Table 1
SOME ADVANTAGES OF TRANSDERMAL MEDICATION

Bypass hepatic ''first pass'' and gastrointestinal incompatibility
Reduce side effects due to the optimization of the blood concentration-time profile
Provide predictable and extended duration of activity
Greater patient compliance due to the elimination of multiple dosing schedules
Enhance therapeutic efficacy
Reduce frequency of dosage
Reversibility of drug delivery which would allow for removal of the drug source
Minimize inter- and intrapatient variation
Self administration

for the patient to be treated for 10 to 14 days.[2] He found that an initial injection of 7 mg/ kg followed by 32 subsequent injections of 5 mg/kg at 10-hr intervals was required. If 14- mg/kg injections were given to reduce the number of injections needed, an effective level could be maintained, but for 8 hr, the concentration of the drug was at a potentially toxic level. If a transdermal controlled release product were available, a single administration providing the 5 mg/kg would be needed.

In Figure 1, the ideal transdermal controlled release rate is illustrated, i.e., a constant concentration, one that is effective but not toxic, is maintained for the desired time. Advantages of this system for therapeutic agents are (1) reproducible and prolonged constant delivery rate, (2) convenience of less frequent administrations, and (3) reduced side effects because the dose does not exceed the toxic level.

B. Advantages and Limitations
1. Advantages
The advantages of transdermal medication indicated above are indeed great. However, transdermal systems can impart other important advantages to active agents that could be sufficient to elevate many products to commercial successes. Table 1 lists a number of these successes, the most important of which are discussed later.

Table 2
RESEARCH EXPENDITURE AND DEVELOPMENT PRODUCTIVITY IN U.S. PHARMACEUTICAL INDUSTRY[3]

	1960	1965	1975
Research expenditure (in million dollars)	200	351	1028
Development productivity (number of new drug entities successfully developed and marketed)	50	25	15
Research & Development effectiveness:			
Cost (million dollars/new drug entity)	2	14	68
Time (years)	2	—	10—15

From Katz, M., *Drug Cosmet. Ind.*, 40, 1980. With permission.

Table 3
THE BIRTH PANGS OF A NEW DRUG[3] (U.S. PHARMACEUTICAL INDUSTRY IN 1970)

	Drug substances
Results from extraction, isolation and synthesis for therapeutic purposes	126,060 (100%)
Submission for pharmacology testing	703,900 (558%)
Selection for clinical testing	1,013 (0.8%)
NDA approval	16 (0.013%)

From Katz, M., *Drug Cosmet. Ind.*, 40, 1980. With permission.

a. Economic Considerations

The cost of developing new drug entities as well as the time it takes to bring such drugs to the marketplace has been continuously increasing, as shown in Table 2.

Thus, in 1975 over one billion dollars was spent in pharmaceutical research and it took an average of 10 to 15 years and over 60 million dollars to bring a new drug to the market.[3] As it is shown in Table 2 in 1960, it took only 2 years to bring a new drug to the marketplace with a research effort of less than 2 million dollars.

Even more startling are the data shown on Table 3 which indicate that while 126,000 drug substances were investigated in 1970, only 16 were approved by the FDA for use on humans that same year; pharmacological and clinical testing and undoubtedly marketing considerations eliminated all other.

In transdermal delivery you may start with a drug that is already approved, therefore, the risks, time to the marketplace, and the research costs are all substantially reduced. These costs will vary from organization to organization but should not exceed 4 million dollars and 4 years.

b. Clinical Improvements

Transdermal delivery can increase the therapeutic value of many drugs by obviating specific problems associated with the drug. Such problems might include, gastrointestinal irritation, low absorption, decomposition due to hepatic "first pass" effect, formation of metabolites that cause side effects, and short half-life necessitating frequent dosing. In transdermal medication, the above problems can be eliminated because the drug diffuses over a prolonged period of time directly into the bloodstream. An excellent example is that of nitroglycerin used in angina pectoris patients as a vasodilator. Nitroglycerin has a 90% hepatic "first pass" effect, so it could not be used orally to prevent angina pectoris attacks. Its main use was as a sublingual pill to abort an attack after it occurred. With the advent of transdermal medication, nitroglycerin is now used as a patch to prevent angina pectoris attacks.

A gold mine might exist in the files of major drug companies in drug substances discarded because of gastrointestinal irritation, low absorption, or other specific problems which can be bypassed by the use of transdermal medication.

2. Limitations

Though the advantages of transdermal medication are impressive, the merits of each application have to be examined individually, and the positive and negative effects weighed carefully before large expenditures for developmental work are committed.

Only a small percentage of the drugs can be delivered transdermally due to three limitations, difficulty of permeation through human skin, skin irritation, and clinical need.

In addition to its use as a physical barrier, the human skin functions as a chemical barrier as well. The outermost layer of the skin, the stratum corneum, is an excellent barrier to almost all chemicals including drugs. The anatomy and biochemistry of skin are discussed in Chapter 3. Thus, if the drug dosage required for therapeutic value is more than 10 mg per day, the delivery transdermally will be very difficult if not impossible. Daily dosages of less than 5 mg are preferred.

Skin irritation or contact dermatitis of excipients and enhancers of the drug used to increase percutaneous absorption is another major limitation. Contact irritant dermatitis results from direct toxic injury to cell membranes, cytoplasms, or nuclei. Contact allergic dermatitis involves host immunological activity. Cutaneous toxicology and testing methodology are discussed in Chapter 13.

Clinical need is another area that has to be examined carefully before a decision is made to develop a transdermal product. Oral medication is adequate for the delivery of most drugs. However, with the recent FDA approval of a 7-day clonidine patch, the clinical need might come in the form of convenience and greater patient compliance due to the elimination of multiple dosing schedules.

III. SYSTEMS FOR TRANSDERMAL DELIVERY OF MEDICATION

The major parts of a transdermal system are

1. A controlled release device comprised of polymers, the drug, excipients, and enhancers.
2. A fastening system, usually a pressure sensitive adhesive, for adhering the device to the skins.
3. A hermetically sealed package composed of impervious films.

A. Brief Description of Controlled Release Devices

Table 4 categorizes the various controlled release technologies including physical as well as chemical systems.[4] The chemical systems do not appear to be useful for the delivery of drugs transdermally. The four major classes of physical systems are described below.

1. Reservoir Devices with Rate-Controlling Membrane

These include microcapsules, macrocapsules, and membrane systems. Membrane systems are most applicable in transdermal delivery and are composed of a liquid containing the drug encapsulated by a solid or microporous polymeric membrane. Such systems are discussed in Volume II, Chapter 5.

2. Reservoir Devices without Rate-Controlling Membrane

These systems include hollow fibers, impregnation in porous plastics such as MPS® porous

Table 4
CATEGORIZATION OF POLYMERIC SYSTEMS FOR CONTROLLED RELEASE

Physical systems
  Reservoir systems with rate-controlling membrane
    Microencapsulation
    Macroencapsulation
    Membrane systems
  Reservoir systems without rate-controlling membrane
    Hollow fibers
    Poroplastic® and Sustrelle® ultramicroporous cellulose triacetate
    Porous polymeric substrates and foams
  Monolithic systems
    Physically dissolved in nonporous, polymeric, or elastomeric matrix
      Nonerodible
      Erodible
      Environmental agent ingression
      Degradable
    Physically dispersed in nonporous, polymeric, or elastromeric matrix
      Nonerodible
      Erodible
      Environmental agent ingression
      Degradable
  Laminated structures
    Reservoir layer chemically similar to outer control layers
    Reservoir layer chemically dissimilar to outer control layers
  Other physical methods
    Osmotic pumps
    Adsorption onto ion-exchange resins
Chemical systems
  Chemical erosion of polymer matrix
    Heterogeneous
    Homogeneous
  Biological erosion of polymer matrix
    Heterogeneous
    Homogeneous

PVC sheet, Millipore® filters, and Celgard® porous polypropylene, foams, and possibly hydrogels and ultramicroporous cellulose triacetate.

The simplest example is perhaps the hollow fibers which hold the active agent in their bore and release it by diffusion through the air layer above the agent. Systems utilizing impregnated porous plastics (PVC and Celgard®, etc.) are more complex, but in all cases, the active agent is retained by capillary action physically imbedded in the pores. Release also occurs by diffusion through the air layer above the liquid that fills the pores. Strictly speaking, most of these systems may be considered monolithic matrix systems, except that interaction of active agent and polymer is minimal. Transdermal devices using ultramicroporous cellulose triacetate are discussed in Volume III, Chapter 4 .

3. Monolithic Systems

Probably the simplest and least expensive way to control the release of a drug is to disperse it in an inert polymeric matrix. In monolithic systems, the active agent is physically blended with the polymer powder and then fused together by compression molding, injection molding, screw extrusion, calendering, or casting,[5] all of which are common processes in the plastics industry.

Similarly, the active agent can be blended with elastomeric materials in the mixing step like any of the other additives, e.g., accelerators, reinforcing pigments, stabilizers, and processing aids.[6]

In both of the above cases, the active agent dissolves in the polymeric or elastomeric matrix until saturation is reached. Any additional active agent, remains dispersed within the polymer matrix, and the system is physically dispersed. As the agent is removed from the surface of the monolithic device, more of the agent diffuses out from the interior to the surface in response to the decreased concentration gradient leading to the surface. Such transdermal devices are discussed in Volumes II and III.

If the polymer is plasticizable or swellable by an environmental agent such as water, the system involves ingression of an environmental agent into the device which plasticizes the polymeric matrix, thereby allowing the physically bound active ingredient to diffuse out.

4. Laminated Structures

In this system, at least two and usually three polymeric films are adhered or laminated together. The center layer of a three-layer laminate is the reservoir layer. It contains a large amount of the active agent and may be made of porous or nonporous polymeric material. The outer layers control the rate of release of the agent and are usually fabricated from a more rigid polymer than that of the reservoir. Should the reservoir layer and the outer films both be made of the same polymer, it is apparent that the system reverts to a monolithic matrix system. A discussion of its ramifications, as they relate to transdermal delivery, is presented in Volume III, Chapter 2.

B. Release Characteristics of Controlled Release Devices

Of the different technologies listed in Table 4, all of the physical processes are in one way or another controlled by the diffusion of the active agent through a polymer barrier or by an inward diffusion of an environmental fluid in the case of "environmental agent ingression" devices and some homogeneous "retrograde chemical reaction" devices. Chapter 2 discusses, in detail, the diffusion of drugs through polymers.

The active agent passes through the polymer or polymeric barrier in the absence of pores or holes by a process of absorption, solution, and diffusion down a gradient of thermodynamic activity until desorbed or removed. The transport of the active agent is governed by Fick's first law:

$$J = \frac{dM_t}{Adt} = \frac{-Dd\ C_m}{dx} \tag{1}$$

where J is the flux in $g/cm^2/sec$, C_m is the concentration of active agent in the polymeric membrane in g/cm^3, dC_m/dx is the concentration gradient, D is the diffusion coefficient of the active agent in the polymeric membrane in cm^2/sec, A is the surface area through which diffusion takes place in cm^2, M_t is the mass of agent released, and dM_t/dt is the steady-state release rate at time t.

Equation 1 can be integrated under the proper boundary conditions for each of the systems listed in Table 4 to obtain an equation giving the amount of agent released as a function of time. In many situations, however, the mathematics become rather complicated, and no explicit equations can be derived. The mathematics of diffusion have been discussed elsewhere.[7-9] However, release characteristics encountered with the most common controlled release systems are mathematically described below.

1. Reservoir Systems with Rate-Controlling Membrane

When applied to these systems, Fick's law predicts that a steady state will be established with the release rate being constant and independent of time if an active agent is enclosed within an inert polymer membrane and concentration of the agent is maintained constant

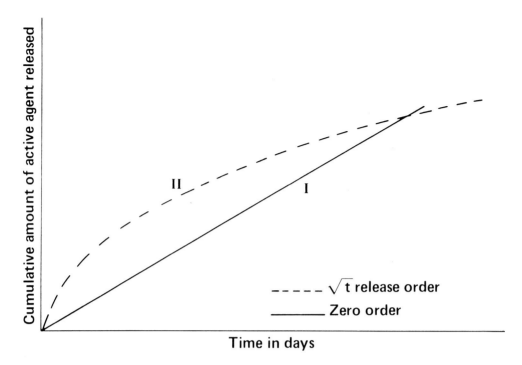

FIGURE 2.   Representation of "zero order" and "$\sqrt{t}$ order" release.

within the enclosure. The amount of active agent released per day is therefore constant for the life of the device, and

$$M_t = kt \tag{2}$$

where k is a constant. The above applies for all geometries of the device, e.g., spheres, slabs, etc. This type of release is "zero order" and is shown as Curve I in Figure 2.

2. Reservoir Systems without Rate-Controlling Membrane

It can be shown that these devices should follow a rate of release proportional to $t^{-1/2}$. The amount of agent released is then proportional to $t^{+1/2}$ ($t^{+1/2}$ order), and given by the equation:

$$M_t = k\, t^{+1/2} \tag{3}$$

This equation gives a parabolic curve as shown by Curve II in Figure 2. With this system, a large amount of the agent is released initially, and substantially smaller and decreasing amounts are released during the last half of the life of the device.

3. Monolithic Systems

Physically dissolved, nonerodible, polymeric, or elastomeric matrix — Release rate in this system is proportional to $t^{-1/2}$, (same as Equation 3) until about 60% of the active agent is released. The release rate thereafter is related exponentially to time, i.e.,

$$\frac{dM_t}{dt} = k_1 e^{-k_2 t} \tag{4}$$

where k_1 and k_2 are constants.

Thus, the rate of release above 60% drops exponentially. This type of release, which is called "first order", is also observed in reservoir systems in which the solution of active agent within the enclosure is less than saturated.

Physically dispersed, nonerodible, polymeric, or elastomeric matrix — The amount released in these systems is proportional to the $t^{+1/2}$ as long as the concentration of the active agent present (dispersed and dissolved) is higher than the solubility of the agent in the matrix. Thus, the dispersed systems are similar to the dissolved systems, except that, instead of a decreased release rate after 60% of the chemical has been emitted, the relationship holds almost over the complete release curve.

4. Laminated Structures

Two cases are easily discernible; first, if the distribution coefficient of the active agent between the reservoir layer and the barrier membrane is much smaller than unity, the system approximates "zero order" release (reservoir system with rate-controlling membrane), and the amount released per day is independent of time.[10] If the distribution coefficient is close to unity, the system approximates the $t^{+1/2}$ order release (monolithic, physically dispersed system).

C. Basic Components of Transdermal Devices

The components of transdermal devices include (1) the polymer matrix or matrices that regulate the release of the drug, (2) the drug, and (3) enhancers and other excipients.

1. Polymer Matrix

Advances in controlled release technology have been rapid because polymer science has become sophisticated enough to incorporate into polymers tailor-made properties for each controlled release application. The importance of polymer selection will be appreciated more if one considers the different design criteria that must be fulfilled

1. Molecular weight, glass transition temperature, and chemical functionality of the polymer must allow the proper diffusion and release of the specific drug.
2. The functionality of the polymer should be such that it will not chemically react with the drug.
3. The polymer and its degradation products must be nontoxic or antagonistic to the host.
4. The polymer must not decompose in storage or during the useful life of the device.
5. The polymer must be easily manufactured and fabricated into the desired product. It should allow incorporation of large amounts of active agent without excessively deteriorating its mechanical properties.
6. Finally, cost of the polymer should not be excessive and thereby cause the controlled release device to be noncompetitive.

A list of polymers that could be used in transdermal formulations is shown in Table 5. To date, polymers that have been used in polyvinylpyrrolidone, ethylene vinyl acetate copolymer, porous polypropylene, polyester, and polyvinyl chloride copolymers.

2. Drug

Judicious choice of drug is the most important decision in the successful development of a transdermal product. The criteria for selecting drugs are shown on Table 6.

The important drug properties that affect its diffusion through the device as well as the skin include molecular weight, chemical functionality, and melting point. These as well as other important parameters on transdermal drug delivery are discussed in Chapter 15. A survey of the recent literature is also discussed in Chapter 16, with emphasis placed on the

Table 5
POSSIBLE USEFUL POLYMERS FOR TRANSDERMAL DEVICES

Natural Polymers

Carboxymethylcellulose	Zein
Cellulose acetate phthalate	Nitrocellulose
Ethylcellulose	Propylhydroxycellulose
Gelatin	Shellac
Gum arabic	Waxes-paraffin
Methylcellulose	Proteins
Arabinogalactan	Natural rubber
Starch	Succinylated gelatin

Synthetic Elastomers

Polybutadiene	Hydrin rubber
Polyisoprene	Chloroprene
Neoprene	Butyl rubber
Polysiloxane	Nitrile
Styrene-butadiene rubber	Acrylonitrile
Silicone rubber	Ethylene-propylene-diene terpolymer

Synthetic Polymers

Polyvinyl alcohol	Polyvinyl chloride
Polyethylene	Polyacrylate
Polypropylene	Chlorinated polyethylene
Polystyrene	Polacrylamide
Acetal copolymer	Polyether
Polyurethane	Polyester
Polyvinylpyrrolidone	Polyamide
Poly(*p*-xylylene)	Polyurea
Polymethylmethacrylate	Epoxy
Polyvinyl acetate	Ethylene vinyl acetate copolymer
Polyhydroxyethyl methacrylate	Polyvinylidene chloride

Table 6
CRITERIA FOR THE SELECTION OF DRUGS FOR TRANSDERMAL THERAPEUTIC SYSTEMS

Proper physiochemical properties
   Molecular weight
   Molecular size
   Water solubility
   Oil solubility
   Melting point
Potent drug
Nonirritant to skin
   Irritant dermatitis
   Allergic dermatitis
Clinical need
   Prolonged administration
   Patient compliance
   Reduction in dosage
   Adverse effects to nontarget tissue

Table 7
ENHANCERS IN
TRANSDERMAL
DELIVERY

Lipophilic solvents
  Dimethylsulfoxide
  Dimethylformamide
  2-Pyrrolidone
Surface active agents
  Sodium lauryl sulfate
  Dodecylmethyl sulfoxide
Two component systems
  Propylene glycol-oleic acid
  1-4 Butane diol-linoleic acid

effect of drug structure on skin penetration. The above-mentioned work indicates that drugs which are efficacious at only a few milligrams per day should be considered for transdermal delivery.

The same results are obtained when one uses the mathematical models developed to predict the permeability of drugs through skin (see Chapter 8). These models are based on the hypothesis that the stratum corneum is composed of parallel and continuous polar and lipophilic pathways, as well as a multilaminate of lipophilic and hydrophilic layers.

Although diffusion of the drug in adequate amounts to produce a satisfactory therapeutic effect is of paramount importance, other parameters such as skin irritation and clinical need should be considered before a drug is chosen as a candidate for transdermal medication.

The drug should, of course, be nonirritating and nonallergenic to human skin. There is very little that can be done if a drug is a strong irritant. The use of prodrugs, discussed in Volume II, Chapter 3, can be used to alleviate this problem in some cases. Prodrugs can also be used to reduce the melting point and change the partition coefficient of drugs so as to increase the permeation through the skin. Unfortunately, the FDA considers prodrugs as new drugs, therefore if such work is undertaken to improve the transdermal chances of success of a drug it should be undertaken early in the life of the drug.

3. Enhancers and Excipients

Enhancers and other excipients which promote skin permeation have to be considered as an integral part of most transdermal formulations because of the excellent barrier properties of the stratum corneum. Enhancers have been classified in three categories as shown in Table 7.

Lipophilic solvents have been found to increase permeation of lipophilic drugs. Dimethylsulfoxide as well as other solvents have been found to be excellent permeation enhancers, possibly because they affect the continuous lipophilic pathway of the stratum corneum.

Surface active agents have also been found to enhance permeation and especially of hydrophilic drugs. Surface active agents are, however, skin irritants, therefore a balance between permeation enhancement and irritation has to be considered if any success can be expected when using these chemicals.

Finally, two component systems have been shown to be very effective permeation promoters. These systems are comprised of a hydrophilic molecule such as propylene glycol and a lipophilic molecule such as oleic acid. It has been hypothesized that these systems affect the multilaminate hydrophilic-lipophilic layers as well as the continuous pathways. The literature and theory of enhancers has been presented in Chapter 9 . In addition, Volume II, Chapter 8 discusses in detail a specific enhancer Azone®, which has been studied with many devices and drugs and has been found to be of interest.

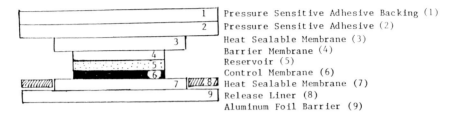

a. Transdermal system with face adhesive.

Barrier membrane (1)
Reservoir (2)
Control Membrane (3)
Pressure Sensitive Adhesive (4)
Release Liner (5)

Pressure Sensitive Adhesive Backing (1)
Pressure Sensitive Adhesive (2)
Heat Sealable Membrane (3)
Barrier Membrane (4)
Reservoir (5)
Control Membrane (6)
Heat Sealable Membrane (7)
Release Liner (8)
Aluminum Foil Barrier (9)

b. Transdermal system with peripheral adhesive.

FIGURE 3.   Schematic diagrams of transdermal systems with (a) face adhesive, and (b) peripheral adhesive.

In the commercial transdermal products, no claims for the usage of enhancers have been made. However, many excipients have been used which I am sure have facilitated the permeation of the drug. Such excipients include: water, propylene glycol, glycerol, ethanol, silicone fluids, and isopropyl palmitate. The effect of hydration, pH, solvents, and other physicochemical parameters are discussed in Volume II, Chapter 4.

D. Adhesives and Packaging

The fastening of all transdermal devices to the skin has so far been done by using a pressure sensitive adhesive. The pressure sensitive adhesive can be positioned on the face of the device or in the back of the device and extending peripherally as shown in Figure 3.

Both adhesive systems have to fulfill the following requirements:

1. Will not cause irritation, sensitization, or imbalance in the normal skin flora during its time in contact with the skin
2. Will adhere to skin aggressively during the dosing interval, resisting the normal spectrum of external insults such as bathing, clothing abrasion, and exercise
3. Will be easily removable without leaving an unwashable residue
4. Will have excellent (intimate) contact with the skin at a macroscopic and microscopic level

In addition to the above, the face adhesive system will have to fulfill the additional requirements:

1. Will be physically and chemically compatible with the drug it is designed to deliver as well as with excipients and enhancers used in the device
2. Will not affect the permeation of drug which should be controlled by the control membrane of the device
3. Will allow the delivery of simple or blended percutaneous absorption enhancers
4. The adhesive properties will not deteriorate as the drug, enhancers, and excipients permeate into the adhesive

The peripheral adhesive system is perhaps less elegant than the face adhesive system and certainly substantially larger. It contains several more layers than the face adhesive system

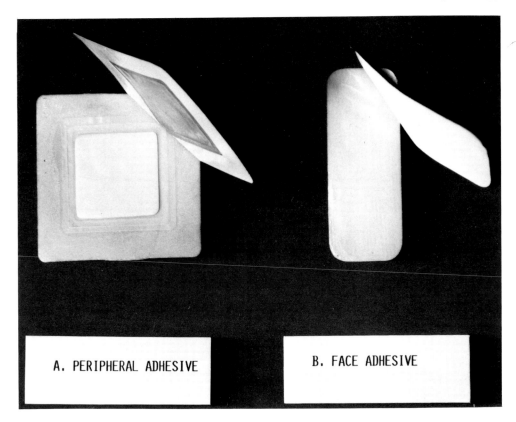

A. PERIPHERAL ADHESIVE

B. FACE ADHESIVE

FIGURE 4.   Photographs of two transdermal products. To the left is a nitroglycerin patch with peripheral adhesive, and to the right an antiasthmatic patch with face adhesive. In both patches the release liner is peeled off to expose the device containing the drug. (Courtesy of the Hercon Division, Health-Chem Corporation.)

and should be more difficult to manufacture. However, there is no need to further package the reservoir layer with the drug. The reservoir of the face adhesive system cannot be hermetically contained, therefore it has to be packaged in an aluminum foil pouch.

Figure 4 is a photograph of two transdermal products, one with peripheral and one with a face adhesive.

IV. SOME COMMERCIAL APPLICATIONS

Though transdermal drug delivery is still a young science, much has been accomplished as indicated by the number of transdermal products that have become commercially available since the first product was introduced in 1981. In Table 8, some information on the commercially available products is shown.

Some of the products are based on monolithic controlled release devices and others on reservoir devices with controlling membrane. The delivery of nitroglycerin from three commercial products is controlled by the skin,[11] but the delivery of scopolamine and clonidine is controlled by the transdermal device.

Another product is expected to receive FDA approval in the near future, an estradiol product by Ciba Geigy. Several other products are under development, including: isosorbide dinitrate, Inderol®, chlorpheniramine maleate, indomethacin, timolol, and a prostaglandin.

Table 8
COMMERCIAL TRANSDERMAL PRODUCTS

Product name	Active agent	Duration (days)	Polymer	Adhesive	Company
Transderm® Scop	Scopolamine	2	Ethylene vinyl acetate	Face	Alza, Ciba
Transderm® Nitro	Nitroglycerin	1	Polypropylene	Face	Alza, Ciba
Nitrodur®	Nitroglycerin	1	Polyvinyl alcohol polyvinyl pyrrolidone	Peripheral	Key
Nitro Disk®	Nitroglycerin	1	Silicone	Peripheral	G. D. Searle
Catapres TTS (Therapeutic Transdermal System)	Clonidine	7		Face	Boehringer-Inglehein
NTS™ Transdermal System	Nitroglycerin	1	Polyvinyl chloride copolymer	Peripheral	Hercon Div. Health-Chem.

REFERENCES

1. **Robinson, J. R.,** Controlled release pharmaceutical systems, in *Chemical Marketing and Economics Reprints,* Long, F. W., O'Neill, W. P., and Stewart, R. D., Eds., American Chemical Society, Washington, D.C., 1976, 212.
2. **Cowsar, D. R.,** Introduction to controlled release, in *Controlled Release of Biologically Active Agents,* Vol. 47, Tanquary, A. C. and Lacey, R. E., Eds., Plenum Press, New York, 1974, 1.
3. **Katz, M.,** The birth pangs of a new drug, *Drug Cosmet. Ind.,* p.40, 1980.
4. **Kydonieus, A. F.,** Fundamental concepts of controlled release, in *Controlled Release Technologies,* Kydonieus, A. F., Ed., CRC Press, Boca Raton, Fla., 1980, 7.
5. **Harris, F. W.,** Preparation of plastic, controlled release, pesticide formulations, in *Proceedings of Controlled Release Pesticide Symposium,* Cardarelli, N. F., Ed., University of Akron, Ohio, 1976, 1, 33.
6. **Cardarelli, N. F.,** Compounding methods for controlled release elastomers, in *Proceedings of Controlled Release Pesticide Symposium,* Cardarelli, N. F., Ed., University of Akron, Ohio, 1976, 1, 44.
7. **Baker, R. W. and Lonsdale, H. K.,** Membrane-controlled delivery systems, in *Proceedings of Controlled Release Pesticide Symposium,* Cardarelli, N. F., Ed., University of Akron, Ohio, 1974, 40, 1.
8. **Crank, J. and Park, G. S.,** *Diffusion in Polymers,* Academic Press, New York, 1968.
9. **Crank, J.,** *The Mathematics of Diffusion,* Oxford University Press, London, 1956.
10. **Kydonieus, A. F.,** The effect of some variables on the controlled release of chemicals from polymeric membranes, in *Controlled Release Pesticides,* ACS Symposium Series 53, Scher, H. B., Ed., American Chemical Society, Washington, D.C., 1977, 152.
11. **Chien, Y. W., et al.,** Comparative controlled skin permeation of nitroglycerin from marketed transdermal delivery systems, *J. Pharm. Sci.,* 8, 968, 1983.

Chapter 2

DIFFUSION THROUGH POLYMERS

Nikolaos A. Peppas

TABLE OF CONTENTS

I. INTRODUCTION

The development of transdermal systems requires judicious selection of a polymeric material or a series of polymers whose diffusive characteristics will be such that a desirable permeation rate of a specific drug or other bioactive agent can be obtained. Therefore, understanding of diffusion in polymers and the mechanisms of drug transport through them is important in controlled release analysis.

In general, the transport mechanism (Fickian or other) establishes the type of solute release. In addition, the solute size and polymer structure control the solute diffusion coefficient, and therefore, the magnitude of the solute release rate.[1-3] In transdermal systems release occurs by molecular diffusion and very rarely by convection.

Molecular diffusion of a drug is related to the molecular size and the polarity of the drug, its solubility in the polymer phase, and the structure of the polymer.

Polymers used in transdermal delivery are usually in the form of thin polymeric films or membranes with or without microscopic pores. From a transport analysis point of view, it is convenient to classify these polymeric films and membranes into three categories.[4]

1.   **Macroporous films and membranes** — These are systems with large pores of average diameter between 0.1 and 1.0 μm. The pore pathway is tortuous and irregular and convective transport may be observed. The morphological characteristics of the polymer are of minor importance in the permeation process of drugs, which is controlled mainly by the size and distribution of pores and the tortuosity of the porous network.

2.   **Microporous films** — These systems have smaller pores usually of diameter between 100 and 500 Å, sometimes as high as 1 μm. The pore structure is again the main parameter influencing permeation of drugs, but drug adsorption on the pore walls and the relative size of drug and pores make the polymer an important factor in the overall process.

3.   **Nonporous films and membranes** — Nonporous films and membranes can be used for a variety of transdermal applications. The polymer films have ''pores'' of molecular size, usually between 10 and 100 Å. Effectively, the spacing between macromolecular chains of the polymer, otherwise known as the ''mesh size'', becomes the controlling factor of controlled release of drugs.[5,6] The polymer structure and morphology are extremely important in achieving a desirable controlled release rate. There are two types of nonporous membranes and polymeric films that are examined in this category, gel membranes, which are polymeric networks swollen in water, and elastomeric membranes, which do not contain any swelling agent.

II. DIFFUSION AND PERMEATION IN MACROPOROUS AND MICROPOROUS POLYMERS

Permeation of drugs through porous polymers is essentially a process which is related to the nature of the porous network available and the tortuosity of the system. The polymer structure plays only a minor role in this process, especially for macroporous membranes, and becomes important only in situations where the drug exhibits strong interactions with the polymer.

A. Prediction of Drug Diffusion Coefficient

Essentially, the process of permeation through porous systems is one involving transport of the drug molecule in a medium which consists of pure water or condensed moisture initially, or a dilute solution of drug long after drug release has started.[7] The existence of a porous network presents natural barriers for diffusion, mainly in the form of molecular collisions between the drug molecules and the pore walls.

In general, diffusion through porous membranes may be described by Fick's law in the form of Equations 1 and 2

$$J = -D_{eff} \frac{dc}{dx} \tag{1}$$

$$\frac{\partial c}{\partial t} = D_{eff} \frac{\partial^2 c}{\partial x^2} \tag{2}$$

Here, c is the drug concentration (usually in mol/cm^3, but in pharmaceutical applications also in g/cm^3), J is the flux of drug (expressed as mol/cm^2/sec or as g/cm^2/sec), x is position, and t is diffusion time.

The diffusion coefficient appearing in these two equations is the effective diffusion coefficient of the drug, D_{eff}, which in its most general form[7,8] is expressed as in Equation 3

$$D_{eff} = D_{sw} \frac{\epsilon K_p K_r}{\tau} \tag{3}$$

Here D_{sw} is the drug diffusion coefficient through water (in the water-filled pores), ϵ is the void fraction (porosity), τ is the tortuosity factor, K_p is the partition coefficient of drug between the pore walls (polymer) and the pore (water), and K_r is a restriction coefficient. The term D_{sw} is usually the drug diffusion coefficient in pure water at the temperature of experimentation. This is a reasonable assumption since, in fact, the pores are filled with a drug solution of continuously changing concentration which is rather difficult to determine. The porosity, ϵ, includes the void fraction (as a fraction from 0 to 1) of all the volume of the polymer film which is available to diffusion (open pores). The tortuosity factor, τ, shows the tortuous path of diffusion due to the irregular direction of the pores; it is usually about three and it increases with increasing chaotic nature of the pore network.[7,9] The partition coefficient takes in consideration the possible distribution of drug between the polymer and the water in the pores as a result of the finite solubility of the drug in the polymer carrier. The value of this parameter is greater for water-soluble drugs diffusing through hydrophilic polymer films. Finally, the restriction coefficient is a geometric factor[10] which depends upon the normalized ratio of the drug molecular radius, r_s, and the average pore radius r_p.

Prediction of the effective diffusion coefficient of drugs through porous membranes for transdermal applications using Equation 3 is not without problems. The term D_{sw} is usually available in the literature either at 25°C or at 37°C but it can be transformed to other temperatures by application of the well-known relation (Equation 4), where η is the viscosity of the solution.

$$\frac{D_{sw}\eta}{T} = \text{constant} \tag{4}$$

The porosity may be measured by mercury porosimetry and corrected appropriately for the compressibility of the polymer and mercury (see, e.g., Miller et al.[11]).

The partition coefficient of drug in a polymer may be measured by classical techniques of soaking a polymer carrier in a drug solution of known concentration. For the determination of the restriction coefficient, the average pore diameter may be measured by mercury porosimetry; the molecular radius is tabulated for various solutes.[6,12] For large nonspherical molecules, the shape and dimensions of the bioactive agent molecule must be taken into consideration.[12]

The tortuosity factor, τ, is the most difficult to determine. Several simplified techniques have been proposed in the literature but they are quite erroneous. Probably the best method to calculate τ is from specific pore models, a variety of which is available in the literature.[7] For most of them τ is around factor 3.

B. Other Methods of Determination of D_{eff}

To avoid the complicated methodology involved in the previous analysis, several investigators have offered semiempirical, but accurate, methods of prediction of D_{eff}. Many of these equations were developed for diffusion in porous membranes and can be applied with confidence to controlled release in transdermal systems.

For example, Faxén[13] developed a general expression which has been modified by Renkin[14] and has been applied to describe solute diffusion through microporous membranes.

$$\frac{D_{eff}}{D_{sw}} = (1 - \lambda)^2(1 - 2.104\lambda + 2.09\lambda^3 - 0.95\lambda^5) \tag{5}$$

Here, λ is the ratio of the drug molecular radius, r_s, to the average pore radius, r_p. This equation has been used by many investigators to describe even drug diffusion through nonporous gel membranes.[15]

Colton and his collaboration have offered a simple model, Equation 6, for the diffusion of compact and relatively rigid biomolecules through membranes.[10,16]

$$\frac{D_{eff}}{D_{sw}} = \frac{1}{\tau} \cdot \exp(-2\lambda) \tag{6}$$

In both situations the terms are as defined in Section II.A.

Finally, excellent approximation methods for predicting D_{eff} for microporous membranes are available. They are based on a hydrodynamic analysis of transport of a small spherical solute in cylindrical pores of a membrane. The theory of Anderson and Quinn[17] gives an accurate prediction of the solute diffusion coefficient through microporous membranes, but unfortunately it has never been used in controlled release.

III. DIFFUSION IN NONPOROUS POLYMERS

Permeation of drugs in polymers with molecular size pores occurs by molecular diffusion in the space available between the macromolecular chains of the carrier.[3,18] For cross-linked polymers this space is equivalent to the mesh size of the network, usually characterized by a linear correlation length. For uncross-linked polymers, the available space is formed by the entangled macromolecular chains. Finally, for semicrystalline polymers, the crystallites act on physical cross-links and a characteristic mesh size, ξ, can be defined as well.

The drug diffusion through these membranes and polymeric films may be expressed by Fick's law in its two forms of Equations 7 and 8

$$J = -D_{sm}\frac{dc}{dx} \tag{7}$$

$$\frac{\partial c}{\partial x} = D_{sm}\frac{\partial^2 c}{\partial x^2} \tag{8}$$

Here, D_{sm} is the drug diffusion coefficient through the polymeric membranes which depends on the molecular characteristics of the polymer carrier. This parameter depends on temperature and the concentration of drug as well.

A. Effect on Polymer Structure on D_{sm}

Diffusional processes through nonporous polymers occur through the space not occupied by the macromolecular chains. Any morphological change which leads to increased diffusional barriers causes an associated decrease of the effective diffusional area, probably also associated with decreased macromolecular mobility.[3]

Control of the solute diffusion coefficient may be achieved by controlling the degree of cross-linking, degree of branching, degree of crystallinity, size of crystallites of the macromolecular carrier, and by adding adjuvants which may slow down the diffusional process either due to hindrance of diffusion or due to thermodynamics changes.[5]

1. Degree of Cross-Linking

In amorphous macromolecular networks, an increase in the degree of cross-linking leads to a progressive reduction of the solute diffusion coefficient. Excessive cross-linking may even lead to complete exclusion of the solute. As the cross-linking density increases, the cross-links approach each other and the available area for diffusion (mesh area), decreases. In addition, the mobility of the chains may drastically decrease and the chains create a smaller effective area for diffusion.[19]

Cross-linking may be achieved by chemical or irradiative techniques. Chemical techniques involve methods of cross-linking of polymers in solution. For example, for hydrophilic polymers several difunctional cross-linking agents may be added in small amount to induce cross-linking between two chains by reaction with functional groups of the backbone chains.

Several examples from recent developments of controlled release systems illustrate the importance of cross-linking in solute release behavior. For example, Lee et al.[20] recently developed matrix-controlled release systems by swelling poly(2-hydroxyethylmethacrylate) (PHEMA) in an ethanol solution of ethylene glycol dimethacrylate (EGDMA), a cross-linking agent for PHEMA, and subsequently treating the system with UV light to create a zone of cross-linking polymer on the outer layer of the devices. The ensuing materials were used to release progesterone and other drugs. It was determined that the outer cross-linked layer of PHEMA was the rate limiting zone for diffusional release, and that, depending on the amount of EGDMA added and time of UV exposure, quasizero-order release rates could be obtained over long periods of times. Similar behavior was observed with cross-linked copolymers of PHEMA and methoxyethoxyethyl methacrylate containing similar drugs.[21] Usually, EGDMA is incorporated in small amount (less than 1 wt %). As the amount of incorporated EGDMA increases, there are more cross-links per unit of volume of cross-linked polymer, and therefore, a greater barrier for diffusion. Therefore, the solute diffusion of coefficient should be considerably lower.

Cross-linked copolymers of methyl methalacrylate (MMA), ethyl acrylate (EA), and *N*-vinylpyrrolidone (NVP) have been used for controlled release of erythromycin and erythromycin estolate.[22] Again, the diffusion coefficient of these solutes decreased as the degree of cross-linking, or the amount of added cross-linking agent, glycidyl methacrylate (GMA), increased. In this study an alternative approach was used to present the data, in terms of the equilibrium swelling ratio, Q, in water, defined as the ratio of the volume of the gel to that of the dry sample. Since loosely cross-linked networks swell more readily, increased values of Q signify lower cross-linking. The results of solute release of erythromycin show that for gels with high swelling ratios, i.e., loosely cross-linked polymers, release was faster. Again, the degree of cross-linking was used as a means of controlling the release rate.

Similar studies have been reported for the release of pilocarpine from poly(vinyl alcohol) (PVA) gels[23] and theophylline and albumin from cross-linked PVA systems.[24] In the first study, γ-irradiation was used to achieve desirable cross-linking. In the second study, chemical cross-linking techniques were preferred, such as reaction of an aqueous PVA solution with glutaraldehyde. This type of cross-linking is slightly different from that observed for PHEMA networks. Here the cross-linking agent (dialdehyde) reacts with the hydroxyl groups of PVA forming a short bridge between two chains. Again small amounts of cross-linking agent are used, usually lower than 0.5 wt %. Our studies[24] have shown that the cross-linked structure is instrumental in controlling the release rates of various solutes, especially large ones such as albumin.

The previous studies addressed predominantly water-swollen polymer networks (hydrogels). Cross-linked polymers, however, can be used as carriers for drug release in the unswollen form as well. The classical example are silicone networks, usually poly(dimethyl siloxanes) (PDMS), prepared by the reaction of silanols and subsequent cross-linking in the presence of peroxides. Folkman et al.[25,26] used these materials for release of steroid hormones and other drugs. Roseman[27] established the importance of the partition coefficient of these drugs in the polymer as a means of controlling the release rate. A special type of cross-linking, known as endlinking, requires a reaction of the difunctional agents with functional groups of the polymer especially created only at the two ends of a chain. For example, controlled cross-linking of silicone chains may be achieved by preparing, α,ω-hydroxylated silicone chains. This method, although widely known among polymer scientists, has not been successful in controlled release technology.

Cross-linking techniques, either by chemical compounds or by irradiation, work best with systems which are initially in liquid form (solution) where uniform dissolution of the cross-linking agent can be achieved. Cross-linking in solid form (powders, particle formulations, etc.) is more difficult. However, recently Kaetsu et al.[28] reported the development of controlled release devices by cross-linking polystyrene, poly(methyl methacrylate), poly(vinyl acetate), and poly(vinyl formal) in solid form by using diethylene glycol dimethacrylate (DGDA) as a cross-linking agent, and by irradiation. Chemotherapeutic drugs for cancer were incorporated and released from these systems at controlled rates affected by the degree of cross-linking.

An accurate analysis prerequisite of the degree of cross-linking effect on solute release rate is the determination of the cross-linking degree of polymers by physicochemical techniques. The polymer literature includes numerous techniques which can be used for determination of the degree of cross-linking (in moles of cross-links per cm^3 of polymer network) or the equally important structural characteristic of the average molecular weight between cross-links, $\overline{M}_c$. An experimental technique we have found suitable for determination of $\overline{M}_c$ of most polymer networks is based on equilibrium swelling studies and analysis of the data using thermodynamic polymer network theories; it has been discussed elsewhere.[29]

Some comments must be made about the effect of branching on solute release. It is well known[30] that branching of the backbone chains of polymers affects the solute diffusion coefficient of solutes through polymers in a similar manner to the degree of cross-linking. However, this approach has not yet been used in the development of controlled release systems.

Finally, for uncross-linked polymers, their molecular weight may be important for drug diffusional release. Usually high molecular weight polymers exhibit a great number of molecular entanglements (physical, semipermanent cross-links) which in turn create a barrier for solute diffusion.

2. Degree of Crystallinity

Crystalline regions of polymers are ordered structures of chains of higher density. Therefore, they are usually impermeable to solute and act as barriers for diffusional release of drugs. Crystallinity may be introduced by heat-treatment (annealing) of polymer systems either during the fabrication or later. The ability of polymers to crystallize depends on their chemical structure, hydrogen bonding, etc. Therefore, polymers with bulky group substituents in their backbone chain are more difficult to crystallize than simpler structures such as polyethylene or PVA.

Researchers have not availed themselves of the full potential of crystallization as a method to control solute release from polymer carriers. In one of the few studies reported,[24] it was determined that theophylline release from heat-treated annealed PVA networks was much slower than that from their amorphous (noncrystalline) counterparts. The diffusion coefficient of theophylline decreased drastically with increased annealing time or temperature.

B. Prediction of D_{sm} by Empirical Methods

Several methods exist for the prediction of the drug diffusion coefficient through a polymer by use of a number of polymer characteristics. Some of these methods apply only to swollen polymers, while others are equally applicable to elastomeric and gel membranes.

Several investigators have developed useful correlations between D_{sm} and polymer properties by examining a range of available diffusive data. For example, Davis[31] proposed Equation 9 which has successfully described solute diffusion through gels and many biological membranes

$$\frac{D_{sm}}{D_{sw}} = \exp[-(5 + 10^{-4}M_s)c_p] \tag{9}$$

Here, D_{sw} is the drug diffusion coefficient through water, M_s is the molecular weight of the drug, and c_p is the concentration of polymer in the gel (expressed as grams of polymer per grams of gel).

Another empirical relation expressed by Equation 9 can be safely used for membranes which are swollen in biological fluids.[32]

$$\frac{D_{sm}}{D_{sw}} = \left(\frac{1 - \upsilon}{1 + \upsilon}\right)^n \tag{9a}$$

Here, υ is the polymer volume fraction of the membrane. This equation is not applicable for systems with very small amounts of swelling agent, i.e., when $\upsilon > 0.9$.

Finally, many simple power laws have been proposed[33-35] not only for diffusion through nonporous polymers but also for diffusion in microporous systems. The general form of these power laws is

$$D_{sm} = a \exp(-M_s^b) \tag{10}$$

where M_s is the drug molecular weight and a and b are two constants.

C. Prediction of D_{sm} by Theoretical Methods

More exact expressions of the drug diffusion coefficient are available through the work of Yasuda et al.[36,37] and Peppas et al.[18,38,39] These include expressions with correlative and predictive capabilities which include solute diffusion in gel and elastomeric membranes. In general, their basic conclusions are that the solute diffusion coefficient is proportional to the macromolecular area for diffusion, the term $\exp(-r_s^2)$, where r_s is the molecular radius, and the term $\exp Q$, where Q is the degree of swelling.

IV. FICKIAN AND NON-FICKIAN DIFFUSION

The structural characteristics described before affect the diffusion coefficient of drugs through polymers but do not alter the type of diffusion observed (Fickian). Therefore, drug release from matrix systems of sheet, spherical, or cylindrical geometry will be time-dependent,[1,2] where t is the release time, whether or not the polymer carriers are highly cross-linked or crystalline. Even in those few cases where zero-order release has been claimed, one must note that the drug release rate is time-independent only within a finite (usually short) period of time.

Drastic effects on the mechanism of diffusion of a solute through a polymer may be achieved by employing the relaxational characteristics of polymer chains. Indeed, when a solvent (dissolution medium, e.g., water or biological fluid) penetrates an originally glassy, hydrophilic polymer, a swollen layer is observed close to the polymer/water surface. Within this gel-like phase drug diffusional release is affected by the continuous relaxation of the macromolecular chains. In general, drug release from these polymers is not Fickian but it follows anomalous transport mechanisms.[40,41] Under certain conditions discussed elsewhere[42] it is possible to achieve zero-order (time independent) release rates.

Several systems have been developed recently which exhibit anomalous or zero-order release of drugs or other bioactive agents.[41] Early investigations of these relaxational effects were reported by Good[43] who studied release of triplennamine-hydrochloride from initially glassy (dry) cross-linked PHEMA. In studies by Hopfenberg et al.,[44] different copolymers of ethylene vinyl alcohol (EVA) were employed to release KCl at non-Fickian release rates. Similarly, Peppas and Franson[42] showed the potential of copolymers of HEMA and MMA as carriers for quasizero-order release of drugs, using theophylline as a model solute.

From a formulations point of view perhaps the most interesting study is that of Korsmeyer and Peppas[24] who reported release of biomacromolecules from dry, heat-treated, cross-linked PVA slabs to water. This study shows the potential of combining the effects of macromolecular relaxations, crystallinity, and cross-linking for the development of new systems. In the special case of the systems reported in this study, an intermediate type of solute release (non-Fickian, but not zero-order release) was observed. Technology related to the development of these systems is still in its infancy and more research is needed in this area.

V. THE MATHEMATICS OF DIFFUSION IN POLYMERS

With the exception of certain types of chemically controlled, osmotically controlled, and some porous systems, all other systems work because the bioactive agent can diffuse through the polymer. Therefore, it is important to discuss what type of structural and morphological modifications can be performed on the polymer to control the solute diffusion coefficient.

Indeed, solute diffusion through the polymer membrane film or matrix of diffusion-controlled release systems is described by Fick's law as written in Equation 7 and/or by the alternative form of Fick's law, sometimes also called Fick's second law, as shown in Equation 8

$$J = D_{sm} \frac{dc}{dx} \tag{7}$$

$$\frac{\partial c}{\partial t} = D_{sm} \frac{\partial^2 c}{\partial x^2} \tag{8}$$

In these equations, J is the solute flux (usually in $mol/cm^2/sec$), c is solute concentration (in mol/cm^3, but in pharmaceutical literature also in g/cm^3), t is release time, and x is position normal to the effective area of diffusion for one-dimensional diffusional processes. To assume one-dimensional diffusion when describing diffusional release with Equations 7 or 8, it is required that the geometric shape of the release device be such that end effects are negligible. For example, this restriction requires that for slabs the thickness be much smaller than the other two dimensions (usually aspect ratio of at least 1:20), whereas for cylindrical devices, the length of the cylinder must be at least 20 times larger than its radius.[3,45]

The solute diffusion coefficient, D_{sm} usually in units of cm^2/sec, is the important structural parameter that can be controlled by modification of the polymer structure. In the form of Equations 7 and 8 it is assumed that D_{sm} is independent of solute concentration, c. This is an assumption widely used when analyzing controlled release systems. Its validity is quite questionable. For example, Fujita[46] proposed several expressions describing the dependence of D_{sm} on c. A more accurate expression of Fickian diffusion under these conditions would be

$$\frac{\partial c}{\partial t} = \frac{\partial}{\partial x} \left(D_{sm}(c) \frac{\partial c}{\partial x} \right) \qquad (11)$$

Derivation of appropriate mathematical models from Equations 7, 8, and 11 is readily achieved. In controlled release technology we are interested predominantly in three types of information:

1. The normalized concentration of drug c/c_o, as a function of normalized depth in the device, x/δ, otherwise known as the concentration profile, where c_o is a reference drug concentration at $t = 0$, and δ is the thickness of the (slab) device or in general characteristic length
2. The flux of drug per effective release area, J
3. The quantity of drug M_t, released at time t

For membrane (reservoir)-type devices where the concentration difference across the polymer is quite large and almost constant for a long period of release time, Equation 7 may be integrated over the thickness δ assuming constant J and D_{sm} to give Equation 12

$$J = \frac{D_{sm}K}{\delta} \Delta c \qquad (12)$$

Here Δc refers to the solute concentration difference across the membrane and K is a solubility-type coefficient which is included to account for sometimes significant changes of the drug solubility in the external (solution) phase and in the polymer membrane. The parameter K is known as the solute partition coefficient, it is dimensionless, and it is defined according to Equation 13

$$K = \frac{c \text{ in membrane}}{c \text{ in solution}} \qquad (13)$$

The permeability coefficient of the solute, P, defined according to Equation 14 and expressed in units of cm/sec, is preferred by membranologists to describe the overall permeation of a solute through a polymer.

$$P = \frac{D_{sm}K}{\delta} \qquad (14)$$

Clearly solute permeation, in addition to reasonable values of the diffusion coefficient, D_{sm}, requires that the partition coefficient be high. This requirement translates into important thermodynamic considerations for solute permeation. A bioactive agent will not diffuse through microporous or gel-type membranes or films unless it is thermodynamically compatible with the polymer. Indeed, polar drugs may readily transport through hydrophilic polymers, whereas hydrophobic drugs have very low (commercially unacceptable) permeation rates through the same systems.

An additional implication of Equation 12 is now obvious. Since for the derivation of this equation we assumed that J is constant, due to the almost constant, high value of Δc, membrane (reservoir)-type devices do give release rates which are independent of release time, at least as long as the assumption of constant Δc is valid. It is well-known that reservoir systems exhibit zero-order release. This fact also implies that the quantity of drug released, M_t, is proportional to release time, t.

Solution of diffusional release problems for matrix systems requires solution of the transient diffusion Equations 8 and 11 with appropriate boundary conditions. Solutions for slabs, cylinders, and spheres under different boundary conditions can be found in Crank,[47] and recent reviews by Peppas[3] and Langer and Peppas.[2] An outline of the mathematical steps for obtaining these solutions is presented below.

1. The appropriate form of Fickian diffusion is selected. If Equation 8 is used, one would expect to be able to obtain analytical solutions. If Equation 11 is used, depending on the form of the function $D_{sm}(c)$, analytical or, more typically, numerical solutions can be obtained. The latter requires application of finite differences or similar techniques.
2. The necessary initial and boundary conditions are established. These conditions describe mathematically the experimental conditions of the release tests. For example, if perfect-sink experiments are performed, one may assume that the concentration c is zero at the polymer/water interface at all release times.
3. Equation 8 is solved by standard techniques of solution of partial differential equations and c/c_o is obtained as a function of x/δ and t. For the reference solute concentration, c_o, one usually uses the initial, constant concentration of the solute in the polymer.
4. The flux, J, may be calculated by differentiation of the previously derived expression and evaluation at the polymer/water interface according to Equation 15

$$J = \frac{dM_t}{A \cdot dt} = \left(D_{sm} \frac{\partial c}{\partial x} \right)_{x=0} \tag{15}$$

It is well known that the final form of J as determined by Equation 15 for most common geometries and experimental conditions and for matrix systems is time dependent, i.e., zero-order release cannot be achieved with conventional matrix systems.

A popular form of Equation 15, which is widely used by pharmacists when plotting release data is the approximate solution for release of dissolved drugs from thin slabs under perfect sink conditions, which for short times only is given by Equation 16

$$\frac{dM_t}{A \cdot dt} = \frac{2M_\infty}{A} \left[\frac{D_{sm}}{\pi \delta^2} \right]^{1/2} t^{-1/2} \quad \text{for} \quad \frac{M_t}{M_\infty} < 0.6 \tag{16}$$

This expression predicts that the drug release rate decreases with increasing release time. M_∞ is the amount of drug released at infinite time.

5. The total amount of drug released, M_t, may be calculated as a function of time by integrating Equation 15 over the total (constant) thickness of the polymer.

$$M_t = \int_0^t J dt \tag{17}$$

Again a popular expression may be derived from Equation 16 which can used only under the same assumptions as for Equation 16

$$\frac{M_t}{M_\infty} = 4\left[\frac{D_{sm}}{\pi\delta^2}\right]^{1/2} t^{1/2} \tag{18}$$

This expression is widely used when treating solute release data by plotting the release drug as a function of the square root of release time.

VI. CONCLUSIONS

The polymer structure is important in controlled release of drugs in transdermal applications. The degree of cross-linking, degree of crystallinity, degree of swelling, size of crystallites, and the macromolecular relaxations of the polymer have an important influence on the solute diffusion coefficient. Depending on the type of polymeric film, different theories for porous or nonporous polymers may be used to predict the drug diffusion coefficient.

REFERENCES

1. **Langer, R. and Peppas, N. A.,** Present and future applications of biomaterials in controlled drug delivery systems, *Biomaterials,* 2, 201, 1981.
2. **Langer, R. S. and Peppas, N. A.,** Chemical and physical structure of polymers as carriers for controlled release of bioactive agents: a review, *J. Macromol. Sci. Rev. Macromol. Chem.,* 23, 61, 1983.
3. **Peppas, N. A.,** Mathematical modelling of diffusion processes in drug delivery polymeric systems, in *Controlled Drug Bioavailability,* Vol. 1, Smolen, V. F. and Ball, L. A., Eds., John Wiley and Sons, New York, 1984, 203.
4. **Peppas, N. A. and Meadows, D. L.,** Macromolecular structure and solute diffusion in membranes: an overview of recent theories, *J. Membr. Sci.,* 16, 361, 1983.
5. **Peppas, N. A. and Gurny, R.,** Relation entre la structure des polymères et la libération contrôlée de principes actifs, *Pharm. Acta Helv.,* 58, 2, 1983.
6. **Lustig, S. R. and Peppas, N. A.,** Scaling concepts in controlled release, *Proc. Symp. Controlled Rel. Bioact. Mater.,* 11, 104, 1984.
7. **Peppas, N. A.,** Modelling of drug release from porous polymers, *Proc. Symp. Controlled Rel. Bioact. Mater.,* 11, 94, 1984.
8. **Cunningham, R. E. and Williams, R. J. J.,** *Diffusion in Gases and Porous Media,* Plenum Press, New York, 1980.
9. **Siegel, R. A. and Langer, R.,** Computer models of factors causing slow release of macromolecules from hydrophobic polymer matrices, *Proc. Symp. Controlled Rel. Bioact. Mater.,* 11, 92, 1984.
10. **Colton, C. K., Scatterfield, C. N., and Lai, C. J.,** Diffusion and partitioning of macromolecules within finely porous glass, *A. I. Ch. E. J.,* 21, 289, 1975.
11. **Miller, E. S., Peppas, N. A., and Winslow, D. N.,** Morphological changes of EVAc-based controlled delivery systems during release of water-soluble solutes, *J. Membr. Sci.,* 14, 79, 1983.
12. **Colton, C. K., Smith, K. A., Merrill, E. W., and Farrell, P. C.,** Permeability studies will cellulosic membranes, *J. Biomed. Mater. Res.,* 5, 459, 1971.
13. **Faxen, H.,** Die Bewegung einer starren Kugel langs der Achse eines mit zahrer Flussigkeit gefullten Rohres, *Ark. Mat. Astron. Fys.,* 17, 27, 1923.
14. **Renkin, E. M.,** Filtration, diffusion and molecular sieving through porous cellulose membranes, *J. Gen. Physiol.,* 38, 225, 1954.
15. **Wisniewski, S. and Kim, S. W.,** Permeation of water-soluble solutes through PHEMA and PHEMA crosslinked with EDGMA, *J. Membr. Sci.,* 6, 229, 1980.
16. **Satterfield, C. N., Colton, C. K., and Pitcher, W. H.,** Restricted diffusion in liquids with fine pores, *A. I. Ch. E. J.,* 19, 628, 1973.
17. **Anderson, J. L. and Quinn, J. A.,** Restricted transport in small pores, *Biophys. J.,* 14, 130, 1974.
18. **Peppas, N. A. and Reinhart, C. T.,** Solute diffusion in swollen membranes. I. A new theory, *J. Membr. Sci.,* 15, 275, 1983.
19. **Peppas, N. A. and Lustig, S. R.,** The role of crosslinks, entanglements, and relaxations of the macromolecular carrier in the diffusional release of biologically active materials: conceptual and scaling relationships, *Ann. N.Y. Acad. Sci.,* 446, 26, 1985.

20. **Lee, E. S., Kim, S. W., Kim, S. H., Cardinal, J. R., and Jacobs, H.,** Drug release from hydrogel devices with rate-controlling barriers, *J. Membr. Sci,* 7, 283, 1980.
21. **Cardinal, J. R., Kim, S. H., and Song, S. Z.,** Hydrogels devices for the controlled release of steroid hormones, in *Controlled Release of Bioactive Materials,* Baker, R., Ed., Academic Press, New York, 1980, 123.
22. **Hosaka, S., Ozawa, T., and Tanzawa, H.,** Controlled release of drugs from hydrogel matrices, *J. Appl. Polym. Sci.,* 23, 2089, 1979.
23. **Yamauchi, A., Matsuzawa, Y., Hara, Y., Saichin, M., Nishioka, Y., Nakao, S., and Kamiya, S.,** The use of PVA hydrogels as a drug carrier, *Polym. Prepr., Am. Chem. Soc. Div. Polym. Chem.,* 20(1), 575, 1979.
24. **Korsmeyer, R. W. and Peppas, N. A.,** Effect of the morphology of hydrophilic polymeric matrices on the diffusion and release of water soluble drugs, *J. Membr. Sci.,* 9, 211, 1981.
25. **Folkman, J., Winsey, S., and Moghul, T.,** *Anesthesiology,* 29, 410, 1968.
26. **Folkman, J. and Long, D. M.,** The use of silicone rubber as a carrier for prolonged drug therapy, *J. Surg. Res.,* 4, 139, 1964.
27. **Roseman, T. J.,** in *Controlled Release of Biologically Active Agents,* Tanquary, A. C. and Lacey, R. E., Eds., Plenum Press, New York, 1974, 99.
28. **Kaetsu, I., Yoshida, M., and Yamada, A.,** Controlled slow release of chemotherapeutic drugs for cancer from matrices prepared by radiation polymerization at low temperatures, *J. Biomed. Mater. Res.,* 14, 185, 1980.
29. **Reinhart, C. T., Korsmeyer, R. W., and Peppas, N. A.,** Macromolecular network structure and its effect on drug and protein diffusion, *Int. J. Pharm. Techn.,* 2(2), 9, 1984.
30. **Mears, P.,** *Polymers: Structure and Bulk Properties,* Van Nostrand Reinhold, London, 1965, 313.
31. **Davis, B. K.,** Diffusion in polymer gel implants, *Proc. Natl. Acad. Sci. U.S.A.,* 71, 3120, 1974.
32. **Collins, M. C. and Ramirez, W. F.,** Mass transport through polymeric membranes, *J. Phys. Chem.,* 83, 2294, 1979.
33. **Sarbolouki, M. N. and Miller, J. F.,** On pore flow models for reverse osmosis and desalination, *Desalination,* 12, 343, 1973.
34. **Sarbolouki, M. N.,** A general diagram for estimating pore size of ultrafiltration and reverse osmosis membranes, *Sep. Sci. Technol.,* 17, 381, 1982.
35. **Michaels, A. S.,** Analysis and prediction of sieving curves for ultrafiltration membranes, *Separ. Sci. Techn.,* 15, 1305, 1980.
36. **Yasuda, H. and Lamaze, C. E.,** Permselectivity of solutes in homogeneous water-swollen polymer membrane, *J. Macromol. Sci. Phys.,* B5, 111, 1971.
37. **Yasuda, H., Peterlin, A., Colton, C. K., Smith, K. A., and Merrill, E. W.,** Permeability of solutes through hydrated polymer membranes. III. Theoretical background for the selectivity of dialysis membranes, *Makromol. Chem.,* 126, 177, 1969.
38. **Reinhart, C. T. and Peppas, N. A.,** Solute diffusion in swollen membranes. II. Influence of crosslinking on diffusive properties, *J. Membr. Sci.,* 18, 227, 1984.
39. **Peppas, N. A. and Moynihan, H. J.,** Solute diffusion is swollen membranes. IV. Theories for moderately swollen networks, *J. Appl. Polym. Sci.,* 30, 2589, 1985.
40. **Korsmeyer, R. W. and Peppas, N. A.,** Macromolecular and modelling aspects of swelling-controlled systems, in *Controlled Release Delivery Systems,* Roseman, T. J. and Mansdorf, S. Z., Eds., Marcel Dekker, New York, 1983, 77.
41. **Peppas, N. A.,** Release of bioactive agents from swellable polymers: theory and experiments, in *Recent Advances in Drug Delivery Systems,* Anderson, J. M. and Kim, S. W., Eds., Plenum Press, New York, 1984, 279.
42. **Peppas, N. A. and Franson, N. M.,** The swelling interface number as a criterion for prediction of diffusional solute release mechanisms in swellable polymers, *J. Polym. Sci. Polym. Phys. Ed.,* 21, 983, 1983.
43. **Good, W. R.,** Diffusion of water soluble drugs from initially dry hydrogels, in *Polymeric Delivery Systems,* Kostelnik, R., Ed., Gordon & Breach, New York, 1976, 139.
44. **Hopfenberg, H. B., Apicella, A., and Saleeby, D. E.,** Factors affecting water sorption in and solute release from glassy EVA copolymers, *J. Membr. Sci.,* 8, 273, 1981.
45. **Peppas, N. A.,** Mathematical models for controlled release kinetics, in *Medical Applications of Controlled Release,* Vol. 2, Langer, R. S. and Wise, D., Eds., CRC Press, Boca Raton, Fla., 1984, chap. 10.
46. **Fujita, H.,** Diffusion in polymer-diluent systems, *Fortschr. Hochpolym. Forsch.,* 3, 1, 1961.
47. **Crank, J.,** *The Mathematics of Diffusion,* Oxford University Press, London, 1975.

Chapter 3

ANATOMY AND BIOCHEMISTRY OF SKIN

Donald L. Bissett

TABLE OF CONTENTS

I. INTRODUCTION

Any effort to deliver drugs across the skin requires at least a basic understanding of the anatomy and biochemistry of that tissue. Entire volumes have been written on those topics.[1-3] This writing will be a condensed discussion. Where appropriate, the emphasis will be on the potential impact of discussed skin properties on transdermal delivery of drugs.

II. ANATOMY OF SKIN

The skin is a multicomponent, multifunction organ. Its functions involve interaction with and adaptation to the environment. Specifically, it serves as a chemical barrier, a physical barrier, the site of thermoregulation, and a sensory end organ. Responses and adaptations to environmental insult are key roles. With such a multiplicity of functions, it is little wonder that the skin is structurally very complex. A diagram of the human skin is presented in Figure 1.

A. Dermis

The dermis constitutes the majority of the mass of skin. It is a dense network of fibrous and elastic tissue. It varies considerably in thickness as a function of body site, from 1 mm on the scalp to 4 mm on the back.

A large part of the dermis is composed of fibrous proteins called collagen and elastin. Between these protein fibers is a gel composed of polymeric sugar (glycosaminoglycans), salts, and water. These protein and sugar structural elements are synthesized and deposited extracellularly by a small population of dermal cells called fibroblasts.

The protein collagen, which comprises about three fourths of the dermal dry weight, is the principal component imparting tensile strength to the dermis. Between the bundles of collagen are networks of the protein elastin. When the skin is deformed by external mechanical force, elastin restores the normal structure of the bundles and, thus, of the skin.

The polymeric sugar (glycosaminoglycan, mucopolysaccharide, and "dermal ground substance") is a mixture of anionic polysaccharides. The specific components are chondroitin 4-sulfate, dermatan sulfate, and heparin. This mixture is the environment in which the dermal fibroblasts reside.

In addition to fibroblasts, the dermis also contains mast cells. While the exact role of mast cells is unclear, they appear to function in the initiation and control of inflammatory events such as disease and injury. Granules within the cells release the molecule histamine which initiates inflammation. This release process is called degranulation since the cells are observed to have a diminished content of granules. Additional information will be presented on inflammatory events throughout this chapter.

Embedded within the dermis are numerous structures: blood vessels, lymphatic vessels, nerve endings, hairs, sebaceous glands, and sweat glands. The latter three open directly into the environment at the skin surface. These openings can provide points of entry for topically applied materials, particularly in regions of the body where they are large or numerous, such as the face.

1. Blood Supply

A system of large arteries lies just below the dermis in what is called subcutaneous tissue. The blood supply of the skin, carrying nutrients, comes from arteriole branches of these arteries. These branches give rise to networks of smaller vessels which permeate the dermis and its embedded structures. The vessels become increasingly smaller as the upper dermis is approached. The network does not extend beyond the dermis. A similar network of venous branches, carrying away waste products and probably most molecules delivered topically, drains into the subcutaneous venous arteries.

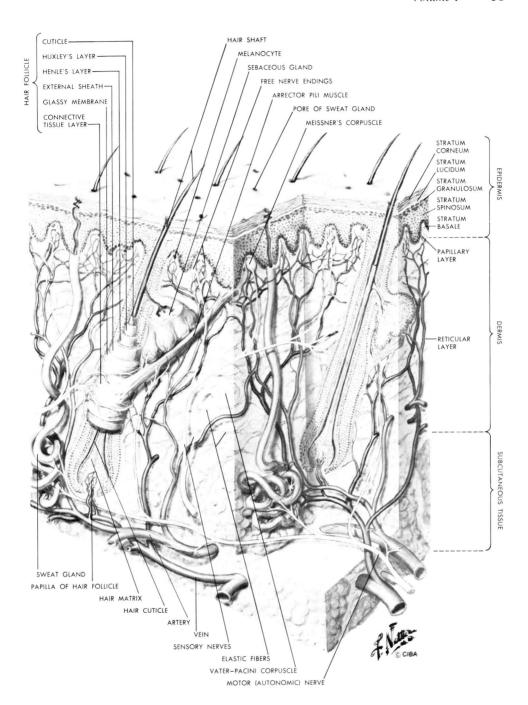

FIGURE 1. Illustration of the structure of skin.(© Copyright 1967, CIBA Pharmaceutical Company, Division of CIBA-GEIGY Corporation. Reprinted with permission from *Clinical Symposia*, illustrated by Frank H. Netter, M.D. All rights reserved.)

Most of the skin circulation is normally composed of microscopic vessels. In response to injury (chemical or physical, stress, disease), these vessels can rapidly dilate, increasing the flow of blood to the site. This flow results, in large part, in the heat and redness of injury. This flow is important in the injured tissue destruction, debris clearance, and tissue repair processes. Specialized inflammatory cells, such as macrophages, leukocytes, and lymphocytes, are released into the tissue to carry out these processes. The intensity of the response is, of course, dependent upon the severity of the injury.

2. Lymphatic System

The lymphatic system arises as terminal bulbs in the upper dermis. The vessels in this system function in the collection and transport out of the skin of particulate and liquid matter from the dermis. Materials transported include inflammatory cells, protein, and possibly topically delivered molecules if they bind to particulates or protein.

3. Nerve Supply

The blood vessels form a network in dermis, as do the sensory nerves. These nerves sense touch, pain, itch, heat, and cold. In contrast to blood vessels, though, the sensory nerves do extend beyond the dermis into the overlying epidermis. There are also nerves which control "motor" functions, such as sweat secretion.

4. Hair and Sebaceous Gland

Hairs are composed of compact cemented cells. They are produced by follicles, which are epidermal appendages extending deep into the dermis. Growing from the sides of the follicles are sebaceous glands. Together, they are called the pilosebaceous units. These units cover all body surfaces except areas such as the palms and soles.

Most hairs grow to a predictable length which is peculiar to a body site. Periodically, hairs are shed and replaced by new hair. This cyclic process is the result of precisely controlled periods of growth and rest of the follicles.

While hair serves an important protective role in most animals, the density of long hair on man is not great enough to serve such a role. Hair is perhaps most important in man as a sensory mechanism. The follicles are surrounded by sensory nerves which respond to any pressure on the hair shaft. This provides a highly sensitive response system.

Hair is composed of as much as 95% protein. Much of the protein is arranged in filaments which are linked by sulfur-sulfur bonds. The principle filament protein is keratin, which has a very high content of α-helical structure. The cross-linked protein structure of hair imparts its great strength.

Sebaceous glands secrete a lipid mixture called sebum into the hair follicle. The sebum then empties onto the skin surface. The gland density on body surfaces where they occur can vary from 100/cm² over most of the body to 900/cm² on the face. The function of sebum in most animals is clearly tied in with the protective role of hair. The low density of human hair argues against such a function in man. Human sebum may have a protective function for the skin surface from some environmental insults.

The composition of sebum synthesized in the glands is shown in Table 1.[4] The skin surface lipids (lipids extracted from the skin surface) differ considerably from sebum for two reasons, contributions from the epidermis and hydrolysis of sebum components by tissue and skin surface microbial enzymes.

5. Sweat Glands

There are two types of sweat glands in the skin, eccrine, and apocrine. They are simple tubular glands, the major portion of them closely coiled deep in the dermis and into the subcutaneous tissue.

The eccrine glands are extremely numerous over the body. The ducts from the glands empty onto the skin surface. These glands function in thermoregulation, responding quickly to heat stress. They eliminate excess body heat, by evaporative cooling, as sweat, a mixture of water, salts, and small organic molecules.

The apocrine glands are much less numerous, present at as little as one tenth the density

Table 1
COMPOSITIONS OF SEBUM AND SKIN
SURFACE LIPID

	% Of component in	
Component	**Sebum**	**Surface lipid**
Squalene	12	10
Sterol ester	<1	2.5
Sterols (unesterified)	0	1.5
Wax esters	23	22
Triacyl glycerols	60	25
Di- and mono-acyl glycerols	0	10
Fatty acids	0	25
Unidentified	5	4

From Nicolaides, N., *Science*, 186, 19, 1984. With permission.

of eccrine glands. They are most numerous in areas such as the underarms, genitals, breasts, head, and abdomen. The ducts from the glands empty into the hair follicle. These glands secrete only a small volume of fluid and are slow to respond to stimuli. The secretion composition varies with body site and can become malodorous perhaps as a result of bacterial decomposition. The function of these glands is not clear.

B. Dermal-Epidermal Junction

The junction of dermis and epidermis is an undulating line of rete ridges (see Figure 2). The pattern varies greatly with body site, being very prominent on the palm and sole but nearly flat in the eyelids.

The junction contains a 500-Å-thick structure called the basal lamina or basement membrane. It is a network of filamentous glycoproteins. Anchoring fibrils extend into the dermis. The membrane appears to serve three functions:

1. Attachment of epidermis to dermis
2. Mechanical support for growth of epidermis
3. Semipermeable filter to transfer of materials/cells across the junction

The basal lamina is not a barrier to small molecules nor probably even to molecules under 40,000 molecular weight. For larger molecules, there is barrier function. However, in tissue injury, the basal lamina becomes very permeable, allowing inflammatory cells to cross and enter the epidermis. There, they function in debris clearance and repair as they do in the dermis.

C. Epidermis

The epidermis is a thin sheet providing the outer covering of the body. It generally ranges in thickness from 0.075 to 0.15 mm, except on the palm and sole where it can be up to 0.6 mm thick. This thin sheet functions as the body's primary protective barrier to environmental insult. Its cells (called keratinocytes for their keratin protein content) undergo a rapid process of division, maturation, and shedding that is unique to skin. Because of the complexity inherent in such a differentiation process, there are many gaps in the knowledge of epidermal functioning, particularly in terms of the controlling mechanisms in differentiation.

1. Basal Cells

Sitting on the dermal-epidermal junction is a one-cell-thick layer of oval-shaped cells,

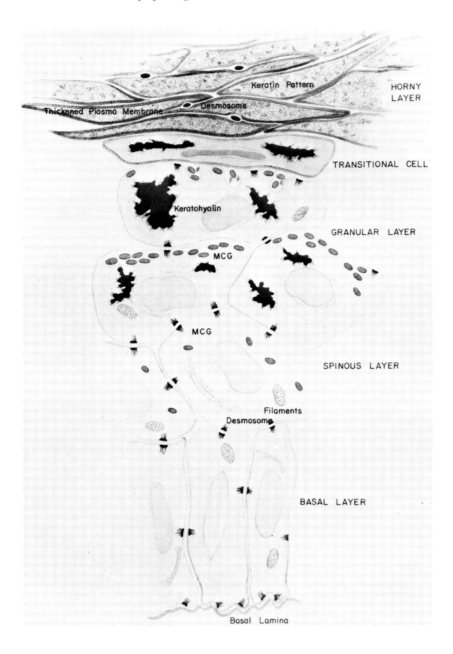

FIGURE 2.   Illustration of the structure of epidermis. (From Montagna, W. and Parakkal, P. F., *The Structure and Function of Skin*, Academic Press, New York, 1974. With permission.)

the basal cells. The cells are much like cells in other body tissues. They have typical intracellular organelles (nucleus, mitochondria, ribosomes, etc.) and possess expected metabolic machinery.

The basal cells are anchored to the basal lamina and to each other by desmosomes. These protein structures occur irregularly on the cell periphery and bridge the gap between cells for attachment. As the cells undergo their process of division and maturation (differentiation), the desmosomes are repeatedly broken and reformed. At all times, though, the cells are in intimate contact with their neighbors.

Mucopolysaccharides are also between cells. They serve as a cell coat or glycocalyx.[5]

The function of this coat is unclear but could be related to cell adhesion, maturation, and cell-cell recognition, among others.

The membranes of basal cells are much like those of other tissue cells; they are rich in phospholipid and cholesterol. The lipids are arranged in a classical bilayer structure with protein molecules embedded in or extending through the membrane.[6] The proteins function in cell adhesion and active transport, among others. (The need for emphasizing this will become clear in the discussion of cell maturation below.)

Within the cells is a complex cytoskeleton of filaments and tubules. These appear to control cell shape and positioning of cell organelles for many of the cell functions. In the epidermis, there is an abundance of keratin filaments within the cytoplasm. These filaments change in composition as the cells differentiate.

In normal skin, the rate of cell production in the basal layer is balanced by shedding at the skin surface. Cells are shed at the rate of one cell layer per day in man. In normal skin, only basal cells divide. When a basal cell divides, on average one daughter cell remains in the basal layer. The other daughter leaves the basal layer and enters the differentiating layers. In injury or disease, mitosis is accelerated and can occur well above the basal layer. The abnormal proliferation is the effort of the tissue to restore a normal epidermal barrier. It can be temporary as in injury, returning to normal with healing. In disease, such as psoriasis, it can be permanent, yielding a constantly inferior barrier.

2. Differentiating Layers

The spinous and granular layers (Figure 2) of cells undergo a rapid differentiation. The spinous cells start as rounded or polyhedral in shape, gradually taking on the flattened shape of a granular cell. Though the nucleus is still present, a spinous cell in normal skin does not divide. In the granular layer, nuclei are absent. (This transformation will be discussed below.)

The spinous cells begin to synthesize specific proteins. This synthesis continues throughout much of the differentiating epidermis. The proteins aggregate into masses called keratohyalin granules.

The keratin filaments of the basal cells aggregate into fibrils. As the cells differentiate, the fibrils elongate, forming an intracellular complex connected to desmosomes on the cell surface. Involved in this fibril formation is a histidine-rich basic protein (filaggrin) synthesized in the granular layer. Filaggrin appears to act as a matrix protein between keratin filaments. Presumably, the keratohyalin granules are the site of the fibril formation.

Also synthesized in the spinous and granular layers are lamellar granules or membrane-coating granules. In the upper differentiating epidermis, these granules migrate toward the cell periphery and their contents are extruded into the intercellular space.[7-9] The contents of the granules are components of the soon-to-be-formed stratum corneum intercellular space and cell envelope.

As cells migrate into the granular layer, intracellular organelles begin to disappear. They are digested by intracellular hydrolytic enzymes released from structures called lysosomes. Organelles such as nuclei, mitochondria, ribosomes, etc. disappear. It is unclear what becomes of all the digestion products but they are probably reutilized in the epidermis for synthesis of other molecules.

The cell membrane also undergoes dramatic changes. The phospholipid content is markedly reduced and ceramides are greatly increased in abundance. Also present is a newly synthesized protein called involucrin which is the protein precursor of the proteinaceous stratum corneum cell envelope.

3. Stratum Corneum (Horny Layer)[10]

While there is a gradual process of change within the spinous and granular layers, there

Table 2
LIPID COMPOSITIONS OF EPIDERMAL LAYERS

Component	% Of component in		
	Basal + spinous	Granular	Stratum corneum
Phospholipid	62	25	0
Sterols (unesterified)	9	21	20
Sterol esters	1	2	2
Ceramides	1	10	52
Glucosyl ceramides	7	8	0
Triacylglycerols	8	2	2
Fatty acids	7	16	22
Hydrocarbons	2	9	0
Others	3	7	2

is a rapid and dramatic transition upon reaching the stratum corneum. It is as if throughout the differentiating layers the stage has been set for this instantaneous event. The transition to stratum corneum can be thought of as a crystallization. (Occasionally in electron micrographs, a transitional cell, a cell intermediate between granular layer, and stratum corneum, is observed. Its rare occurrence limits serious study.)

Stratum corneum cells are extremely elongated and flat (approximately 1-μm thick). They appear stacked in vertical columns in many species and regions of the body. In cross-section, they have a roughly hexagonal shape.[11] Human stratum corneum is 15- to 20-cell-layers thick except on the sole and palm where thicknesses are much greater.

Among the abrupt changes occurring upon reaching the stratum corneum is the intracellular composition. There is an absence of organelles, all having been enzymatically digested in the granular layer. The cell is filled with protein arranged in fibrils. The protein fibrils are composed of keratin and filaggrin. The fibrils appear attached to desmosomes, which at irregular intervals bridge the gap between cells. This complex probably functions as the cell attachment and tissue elasticity element.

In place of the typical plasma membrane (bilayer lipid structure) is a cell envelope. This 100-Å-thick envelope contains a highly cross-linked protein. The cross-links occur between lysine ϵ-amino groups and glutamic acid γ-carboxyl groups of adjacent protein chains. Unlike bilayer lipid membranes, this envelope does not require lipid for structural integrity. The cross-linked protein network is the structural element. In fact, total lipid extraction of stratum corneum does not affect cell or tissue integrity.

Within the cell envelope and between cells is a lipid-rich environment. The intercellular space has been estimated to be 30% by volume of stratum corneum.[12] The lipids (10% of the tissue dry weight) are here, having been extruded there by the lamellar granules. The lipids have a lamellar (layered) structure much like that in the original granules.[7-9] The composition of this lipid is shown in Table 2.[13-16] This stratum corneum lipid composition is ideally suited as a barrier to transport.

In addition to lipid composition changes, element and water profiles change. Phosphorus, sodium, and potassium levels drop 10- to 20-fold in stratum corneum. Levels of other elements, such as sulfur, chlorine, and calcium, remain nearly constant across epidermis.[17] The inner stratum corneum is in contact with a very moist environment, the granular cells. The outer stratum corneum is in contact with a relatively dry environment, the atmosphere. This creates a substantial gradient of water content across the tissue.[18,19]

The cells maintain their general shape and size throughout their residence time in the stratum corneum. They are pushed upward by underlying cells and eventually lost at the skin surface as single cells or small clusters of cells. The cell loss process is called desquamation. The rate of cell loss is approximately one cell layer per day. (In scaling disorders, the clusters of cells lost can be composed of huge numbers of cells. The rate of cell loss can be 10 to 20 times normal.)

The lack of organelles, typical metabolic machinery, and membrane transport systems within stratum corneum cells prompts many to refer to this tissue as dead. However, there are many constants within the tissue, such as thickness, suggesting a regulated system. While the cells do not divide or grow, there is enzymatic activity and control.

The mechanism for desquamation may involve a biochemical (enzymatic) process. Since desmosomes (protein) appear to bind cells together, a proteolytic enzyme is probably involved in desquamation. There is a gradual increase in cell cohesion as a function of depth from the surface.[20] This suggests a gradual loss of cell contact near the surface. However, approximately half-way through the tissue, cell cohesion is very tight. This suggests that the desquamation process begins at the mid-point of the stratum corneum. The mechanisms by which desquamation is initiated and controlled are not known.

Another enzymatic process has also been found to begin in the stratum corneum. Filaggrin synthesized in the granular layer is present as a matrix protein in the lower stratum corneum. However, filaggrin is absent from the upper stratum corneum. It appears to be degraded to amino acids.[21-23] Such a thorough degradation probably requires a variety of enzymes. Coincidentally, along with this degradation is the microscopic observation of loss of protein organization within the cells. Since the intracellular proteins are tied in with the desmosomes, the filaggrin breakdown may be involved in the desquamation process.

4. *Other Cell Types*

There are a variety of other cell types in the epidermis. They include melanocytes, Langerhans' cells, and Merkle cells. Combined, they are a very small percentage of the total cell population. They will be discussed only briefly.

Melanocytes reside among basal cells and synthesize the melanin pigments. The pigments are then transferred to differentiating keratinocytes which retain them throughout their epidermal residence time. In response to ultraviolet light, melanocytes greatly increase their pigment output (tanning). The melanins largely determine skin color and absorb potentially damaging ultraviolet wavelengths.

Langerhans' cells are highly dendritic. The dendrites extend throughout the epidermis. The cells serve a critical role in the immunology of skin, determining response to chemicals in the environment. They may also be involved in other tissue functions.

Merkel cells reside among basal cells and are situated close to nerve terminals in the underlying dermis. They may function in the sensory system.

In skin disease or injury, the cell population in the epidermis can change dramatically. There is an influx of cells associated with inflammation, polymorphonuclear leukocytes (neutrophils), macrophages, and lymphocytes. Their role is destruction of damaged tissue, removal of debris, and repair of the damage. As such, they are generally temporary residents of the epidermis, being cleared eventually by the lymphatic vessels.

D. Tissue Variability

The preceding discussion dealt primarily with normal human skin. Even for normal skin, there is considerable variation among species, among individuals within a species, and among body sites within an individual. For the investigation of skin transport, these variations should be considered in choosing a model system.

Among species, there are differences in tissue thickness, desquamation rate, hair density, gland density, lipid composition, metabolism, etc. There is no perfect substitute for human skin in modeling its properties. However, pig skin is remarkably similar to human skin.[24] It can be used to model many human skin properties.

Among individuals within a species, there are also differences[25,26] as there are among species, although certainly not to the same extent. Additional influences on these parameters within a species arise based on sex, physical health, and age. Marked effects of age include wrinkling, loss of elasticity, reduced blood supply to the skin, thinning of the skin, reduction of the rete ridges, reduction in sebum production, changes in hair growth patterns, etc.[27] The aging of skin involves more than chronological aging. Excessive exposure of the skin to sunlight can dramatically accelerate the skin aging process and result in nonchronological aging events, especially in the dermis.[27-29] Both chronological and solar aging of the skin are poorly understood.

Among body sites within an individual, these same differences can occur.[26] Of particular importance would be the differences in tissue thickness, sebum production, and number of openings (gland ducts and hair follicles) among body sites. Lipid composition among body sites is known to affect transport.[30] The large size and number of openings on facial skin provide ample routes of entry into the body which can complicate analyses of epidermal transport.

E. Responses to Environment

Skin is in direct contact with the environment. It responds quickly and often dramatically to factors in the environment. A few will be discussed here for illustrative purposes.

Scaling skin disorders can greatly alter the normal course of cell division, differentiation, and desquamation in the epidermis. (For the purposes of this discussion, diseases, both genetic and externally induced, will be considered environmental in nature.) The disorders can be confined to the stratum corneum only where desquamation is altered, as may be the case in dry skin. The entire epidermis can be involved with a 10 to 20 times faster rate of cell production and desquamation, as in psoriasis. In the more extreme disorders, immature cells enter the stratum corneum, yielding improper cell stacking, an abnormal lipid composition, and an altered barrier. Each disorder has its particular course of events and effects on epidermal structure and function.

External trauma such as heatburn, sunburn, irritants, and infection dramatically alter tissue activity. There is an immediate local increase in dermal blood circulation to bring in defensive cells and in lymphatic circulation to rapidly carry away the irritant or products of the trauma. There is an influx of specialized cells from the dermis and the dermal circulatory system. The role of this "dermal infiltrate" is to clean up the skin, destroying damaged tissue and removing the debris. There is a delayed burst of mitotic activity in the epidermis to replace the damaged tissue. Temporarily, this will yield a thickened, rapidly differentiating epidermis. Gradually, the system returns to normal.

Not only does the skin respond to the environment but it also adapts to it. Tanning is an easily observed response to exposure to sunlight. Melanocytes produce granules of the pigment melanin. The granules are distributed to the differentiating epidermal cells, which carry them into the stratum corneum. The melanin absorbs ultraviolet light to protect the differentiating epidermis from damage.

Repeated abrasion of skin will result in production of a thickened stratum corneum. Friction surfaces such as the palm and sole commonly produce callus tissue. This thickened tissue acts as a barrier to further mechanical damage of the underlying epidermis.

Skin can also become accommodated to chemical insult.[31] Repeated damage of skin with detergent eventually yields a tissue which no longer is irritated by subsequent exposure. The mechanism of protection here is unknown.

The function of the skin is to protect the body from the environment. As the preceding discussion indicates, it serves this function well. Its remarkable ability to adapt to a changing environment is the key to its success in this role.

III. BIOCHEMISTRY OF SKIN

In common with other tissues of the body, the skin has two metabolic requirements, small molecular weight building blocks for synthesis and chemical energy. Therefore, the basic metabolic machinery of normal skin is much like that found elsewhere in the body. These basic processes will not be discussed here but can be found elsewhere.[32] In addition, there are dissimilarities peculiar to the function of the skin. These peculiarities are most interesting and will be dealt with here, especially as they might impact transdermal drug delivery.

A. Dermis

Protein synthesis (from amino acid precursors) is a key factor in dermal metabolism. Fibroblasts produce and deposit, extracellularly, huge quantities of collagen and elastin. There would appear also to be mechanisms for degradation and replacement of existing protein. This becomes important in repair/turnover of dermal proteins altered by environmental sunlight.[33,34] Extensive protein synthesis also occurs in hair follicles where hair, consisting of approximately 95% protein, originates.

The sebaceous glands produce large quantities of lipid (from the two-carbon precursor acetate). While the classes of lipids are not unusual (Table 1), some of the members within the classes are. The unusual lipids have been discussed by Nicolaides.[4]

These processes require a large energy input. The source of that energy is aerobic carbohydrate (glucose) metabolism. Glucose is delivered by dermal circulation and stored intracellularly as the polysaccharide glycogen. This polymer is hydrolyzed to glucose units as energy is required. It is metabolized to CO_2 and H_2O in the presence of tissue oxygen, also supplied by the dermal circulation. The energy derived from the metabolism is used for cellular synthetic processes.

B. Epidermis

The source of energy for the lower portions of the epidermis is also glucose. However, the glycogen stores are not large. As cells leave the basal layer, they move away from their source of nutrients and oxygen, the dermal blood supply. The system gradually converts to anaerobic metabolism. While the movement away from dermis may not dramatically reduce nutrient and oxygen supplies, glucose and oxygen are no longer utilized extensively for energy. The end product of anaerobic glucose metabolism is lactic acid, which accumulates in skin.[35] Associated with this is a drop in tissue pH from the usual 7 to less than 6.[36,37]

To generate energy for cellular functions, the cells rely primarily on lipids, specifically fatty acids.[38] These fatty acids are derived from the degradation of phospholipids from membranes. The energy derived is used in synthesis of the proteins and lipids for construction of stratum corneum.

During differentiation from basal cells to stratum corneum, the entire cellular make-up changes. A necessary part of this process is degradation of the existing cellular components. Specialized cellular organelles called lysosomes contain a host of lytic enzymes which they release for intracellular lysis. The epidermis is a reservoir of such lytic enzymes.[39-45] Many of these enzymes are inactivated (probably by autolytic processes) in the upper granular layer, however, many also survive into the stratum corneum.[46-50] As discussed previously, the stratum corneum also has proteolytic enzymes, which are probably distinct from granular layer enzymes, involved in desquamation.

C. Skin Surface

The skin surface has a population of microorganisms.[51] They can contribute to the skin enzymology. Their diversity and abundance can vary considerably among individuals and body sites. As mentioned previously (Table 1), they can affect skin surface lipid composition via hydrolysis of secreted sebum.

D. Implications for Drug Transport

The lytic enzyme activity of the skin is probably the most interesting from a drug transport angle. This activity can be advantageous. For materials that do not transport readily, e.g., because of polarity or charge, derivatives can be prepared. For example, an ester derivative (prodrug) might readily traverse the stratum corneum. Within the epidermis, it might be hydrolyzed to the active drug. The derivative would have to be selected to take advantage of enzyme specificities within the epidermis while avoiding premature hydrolysis in the stratum corneum. Hydrolysis in the stratum corneum could negate the advantage of the prodrug for transport enhancement.

The enzyme activity could also be disadvantageous. A drug could be hydrolyzed to inactivate products during transport. A knowledge of tissue enzyme specificities could help in design of hydrolysis-resistant drug actives. A theoretical consideration of skin as a drug metabolizing barrier has been made.[52]

A difficulty in the study of tissue enzymes is appropriate methodology for isolating tissue layers. Methods either employ strong chemical, enzymatic, or heat treatments, which can inactivate tissue enzymes or introduce artifacts. Tape stripping of the skin surface in vivo followed by analyses of the tapes is the method involving the least complications.[46] The limitation is the small quantity of tissue obtained. Skin scrapings[47,48] and thin horizontal sections[49] have also been used.

REFERENCES

1. **Montagna, W. and Parakkal, P. F.,** *The Structure and Function of Skin,* Academic Press, New York, 1974.
2. **Goldsmith, L. A.,** *Biochemistry and Physiology of the Skin,* Vols. 1 and 2, Oxford University Press, New York, 1983.
3. **Mier, P. D. and Cotton, D. W. K.,** *The Molecular Biology of Skin,* Blackwell Scientific, Oxford, 1976.
4. **Nicolaides, N.,** Skin lipids: their biochemical uniqueness, *Science,* 186, 19, 1974.
5. **Fritsch, P., Wolff, K., and Honigsmann, H.,** Glycocalyx of epidermal cells in vitro: demonstration and enzymatic removal, *J. Invest. Dermatol.,* 64, 30, 1975.
6. **Singer, S. J. and Nicholson, G. L.,** The fluid mosaic model of the structure of cell membranes, *Science,* 175, 720, 1972.
7. **Lavker, R. M.,** Membrane coating granules: the fate of the discharged lamellae, *J. Ultrastruct. Res.,* 55, 79, 1976.
8. **Elias, P. M., Brown, B. E., Fritsch, P., Goerke, J., Gray, G. M., and White, R. J.,** Localization and composition of lipids in neonatal mouse stratum granulosum and stratum corneum, *J. Invest. Dermatol.,* 73, 339, 1979.
9. **Wertz, P. W. and Downing, D. T.,** Glycolipids in mammalian epidermis: structure and function in the water barrier, *Science,* 217, 1261, 1982.
10. **Marks, R. and Plewig, G.,** *Stratum Corneum,* Springer-Verlag, New York, 1983.
11. **Menton, D. N.,** A minimum surface mechanism to account for the organization of cells into columns in the mammalian epidermis, *Am. J. Anat.,* 145, 1, 1975.
12. **Elias, P. M. and Leventhal, M. E.,** Intercellular volume changes and cell surface area expansion during cornification, *Eur. J. Cell Biol.,* 22, 439a, 1980.
13. **Elias, P. M.,** Lipids and the epidermal permeability barrier, *Arch. Dermatol.,* 270, 95, 1981.
14. **Gray, G. M., White, R. J., Williams, R. H., and Yardley, H. J.,** Lipid composition of the superficial stratum corneum cells of pig epidermis, *Br. J. Dermatol.,* 106, 59, 1982.
15. **Gray, G. M. and Yardley, H. J.,** Different populations of pig epidermal cells: isolation and lipid composition, *J. Lipid Res.,* 16, 441, 1975.
16. **Yardley, H. J. and Summerly, R.,** Lipid composition and metabolism in normal and diseased epidermis, *Pharmacol. Ther.,* 13, 357, 1981.
17. **Wei, X., Roomans, G. M., and Forslind, B.,** Elemental distribution in guinea pig skin as revealed by X-ray microanalysis in the scanning transmission microscope, *J. Invest. Dermatol.,* 79, 167, 1982.
18. **Wu, M.-S., Yee, D. J., and Sullivan, M. E.,** Effect of a skin moisturizer on the water distribution in human stratum corneum, *J. Invest. Dermatol.,* 81, 446, 1983.

19. **Blank, I. H., Moloney, J., Emslie, A. G., Simon, I., and Apt, C.,** The diffusion of water across the stratum corneum as a function of its water content, *J. Invest. Dermatol.,* 82, 188, 1984.

20. **King, C. S., Barton, S. P., Nicholls, S., and Marks, R.,** The change in properties of the stratum corneum as a function of depth, *Br. J. Dermatol.,* 100, 165, 1979.

21. **Barrett, J. G. and Scott, I. R.,** Pyrrolidone carboxylic acid synthesis in guinea pig epidermis, *J. Invest. Dermatol.,* 81, 122, 1983.

22. **Scott, I. R.,** Factors controlling the expressed activity of histidine ammonia lyase in the epidermis and the resulting accumulation of urocanic acid, *Biochem. J.,* 194, 829, 1981.

23. **Horii, I., Kawasaki, K., Koyama, J., Nakayama, Y., Nakajima, K., Okazaki, K., and Seiji, M.,** Histidine-rich protein as a possible origin of free amino acids of stratum corneum, *J. Dermatol.,* 10, 25, 1983.

24. **Bissett, D. L. and McBride, J. F.,** The use of the domestic pig as an animal model of human dry skin and for comparison of dry and normal skin properties, *J. Soc. Cosmet. Chem.,* 34, 317, 1983.

25. **Anderson, R. L. and Cassidy, J. M.,** Variations in physical dimensions and chemical composition of human stratum corneum, *J. Invest. Dermatol.,* 61, 30, 1973.

26. **Southwell, D., Barry, B. W., and Woodford, R.,** Variations in permeability of human skin within and between specimens, *Int. J. Pharm.,* 18, 299, 1984.

27. **Kligman, A. M.,** Perspectives and problems in cutaneous gerontology, *J. Invest. Dermatol.,* 73, 39, 1979.

28. **Smith, J. G., Davidson, E. A., Sams, W. M., and Clark, R. D.,** Alterations in human dermal connective tissue with age and chronic sun exposure, *J. Invest. Dermatol.,* 39, 347, 1962.

29. **Smith, J. G. and Finlayson, G. R.,** Dermal connective tissue alterations with age and chronic sun damage, *J. Soc. Cosmet. Chem.,* 16, 527, 1965.

30. **Elias, P. M., Cooper, E. R., Korc, A., and Brown, B. E.,** Percutaneous transport in relation to stratum corneum structure and lipid composition, *J. Invest. Dermatol.,* 76, 297, 1981.

31. **McOsker, D. E. and Beck, L. W.,** Characteristics of accommodated (hardened) skin, *J. Invest. Dermatol.,* 48, 372, 1967.

32. **Lehninger, A. L.,** *Biochemistry,* Worth Publishers, New York, 1977.

33. **Kligman, L. H., Che, H. D., and Kligman, A. M.,** Enhanced repair of UV-induced dermal damage by topical retinoic acid, *J. Invest. Dermatol.,* 78, 347, 1982.

34. **Kligman, L. H., Akin, F. J., and Kligman, A. M.,** Sunscreens promote repair of ultraviolet radiation induced dermal damage, *J. Invest. Dermatol.,* 81, 98, 1983.

35. **Smeenk, G. and Rijnbeek, A. M.,** The water-binding properties of the water-soluble substances in the horny layer, *Acta Dermatol. Venereol.,* 49, 476, 1969.

36. **Memmesheimer, A.,** The hydrogen ion concentration of the outer surface of the skin, *Klin. Wochenschr.,* 3, 2102, 1924.

37. **Sharlit, H. and Scheer, M.,** The hydrogen ion concentration of the surface of healthy unimpaired skin, *Arch. Dermatol. Syphilol.,* 7, 592, 1923.

38. **Anastasia, J. V. and Conley, J. P.,** The role of fatty acid oxidation in the epidermis, *J. Invest. Dermatol.,* 69, 430, 1977.

39. **Mier, P. D. and van den Hurk, J. J. M. A.,** Lysosomal hydrolases of the epidermis. I. Glycosidases, *Br. J. Dermatol.,* 93, 1, 1975.

40. **Mier, P. D. and van den Hurk, J. J. M. A.,** Lysosomal hydrolases of the epidermis. II. Ester hydrolases, *Br. J. Dermatol.,* 93, 391, 1975.

41. **Mier, P. D. and van den Hurk, J. J. M. A.,** Lysosomal hydrolases of the epidermis. III. Peptide hydrolases, *Br. J. Dermatol.,* 93, 509, 1975.

42. **Mier, P. D. and van den Hurk, J. J. M. A.,** Lysosomal hydrolases of the epidermis. IV. Overall profile in comparison with dermis and other tissues, *Br. J. Dermatol.,* 94, 443, 1976.

43. **Mier, P. D., Cotton, D. W. K., van den Hurk, J. J. M. A., and Jonckheer-Vanneste, M. M. M.,** Lysosomal hydrolases of the epidermis. V. Horizontal distribution of hydrolases in cow snout epidermis, *Br. J. Dermatol.,* 94, 535, 1976.

44. **Mier, P. D. and van den Hurk, J. J. M. A.,** Lysosomal hydrolases of the epidermis. VI. Changes in disease, *Br. J. Dermatol.,* 95, 271, 1976.

45. **Seppa, H. E. J., Jansen, C. T., and Hopsu-Havu, V. K.,** Proteolytic enzymes in the skin, *Acta Dermatol. Venereol.,* 51, 35, 1971.

46. **Kermici, M., Bodereau, C., and Aubin, G.,** Measurement of biochemical parameters in the stratum corneum, *J. Soc. Cosmet. Chem.,* 28, 151, 1977.

47. **Peter, G., Schubert, E., and Peter, R.,** Biochemical studies on enzyme activities and substrate concentrations in serum and scales of normal subjects and psoriatics, *Biochem. Med.,* 12, 242, 1975.

48. **Forster, F. J., Neufahrt, A., Stockum, G., Bauer, K., Frenkel, S., Fertig, U., and Leonhardi, G.,** Subcellular distribution of phosphatases, proteinases, and ribonucleases in normal human stratum corneum and psoriatic scales, *Arch. Dermatol. Res.,* 254, 23, 1975.

49. **Cotton, D. W. K., Janzing-Pastors, M. H. D., and Jonckheer-Vanneste, M. M. M.,** Horizontal distribution of three dehydrogenases in the cow snout epidermis, *Dermatologica,* 151, 16, 1975.
50. **Roelfzema, H., van den Hurk, J. J. M. A., and Mier, P. D.,** Acid hydrolase activity in normal human callus and in psoriatic scales, *Dermatologica,* 152, 337, 1976.
51. **Sonnenwirth, A. C.,** Bacteria indigenous to man, in *Microbiology,* Davis, B. D., Dulbecco, R., Eisen, H. N., Ginsberg, H. S., and Wood, W. B., Eds., Harper & Row, New York, 1973, chap. 42.
52. **Ando, H. Y., Ho, N. F. H., and Higuchi, W. I.,** Skin as an active metabolizing barrier. I. Theoretical analysis of topical bioavailability, *J. Pharm. Sci.,* 66, 1525, 1977.

Section II: Methods

Chapter 4

IN VITRO TRANSPORT

Gordon L. Flynn, Ward M. Smith, and Timothy A. Hagen

TABLE OF CONTENTS

I. INTRODUCTION

The attainment of an effective concentration of a drug at its active site in a biological system is determined by the physicochemical attributes of the drug as these govern its interplay with all membranes, all phases, and all substances to be encountered between the point of application of the drug and its locus of action. Often, one particular event in the cascade of steps stands out as being of overwhelming importance and, when this event can be singled out and studied, the general scope of the drug delivery problem and the feasibility of delivery of a particular agent can be resolved. The critical, activity-determining event in the case of transdermal delivery more often than not is diffusive passage across the compact outer layer of the skin, the stratum corneum. This is true irrespective of whether the action of a drug is to be local or systemic. Therefore, in vitro techniques of study of percutaneous permeation have formed an important part of research strategies aimed at development of conventional topical dosage forms and newer transdermal systems.

Two distinctly different but in many ways complimentary benchtop approaches have developed in skin permeability research over the years. When it was discovered that skin could be excised apparently without loss in its essential membrane qualities, researchers began placing skin sections in the kind of diffusion cell widely used to obtain exacting mass transfer coefficients for other membranous materials. Diffusion cells for this purpose characteristically have the membrane clamped between and separating two well-stirred fluid phases. The permeation of a chemical from one of the phases to the other is followed carefully and the permeation rate (flux) is determined either from the depletion of concentration of the phase containing the chemical charge (donor phase) or from the accumulating concentration of the chemical in the opposing phase in which it is diffusionally received (receiver phase). If the experimental circumstances are tailored properly the rate can be reduced to a quantitative mass transfer coefficient (permeability coefficient) characteristic of the diffusing chemical, the fluid vehicle phase in which the chemical is applied and, of course, the membrane.

The second kind of diffusion cell alluded to is unique to skin permeation research and is the outgrowth of the experimentalist's desire and attempt to simulate, as closely as possible in an in vitro experiment, the circumstances and conditions under which topical dosage forms actually deliver drugs. In this case, the vehicle is thinly layered over the outer surface of a section of skin in much the same way as it would be spread clinically and diffusion of the drug it contains is followed into a singular, stirred reservoir placed beneath the skin sample. Generally speaking, data from this so-called finite dose diffusion cell or Franz cell do not lend themselves to reduction to characteristic mass transfer coefficients. But, on the other hand, the experimental results give a reasonable picture of how much drug can be induced to pass through the skin barrier in any given fixed time from real formulations. The relative drug delivery merits of different formulations are judged by comparing the results of finite applications of each at a fixed total drug concentration.

It is interesting and instructive to compare the uses to which these different types of cells may be put. The two-reservoir diffusion cell yields quantitative mass transfer (permeability) coefficients. As will soon be evident, relationships of the permeability coefficient to permeant structure for a given membrane and medium of application are insightful with respect to the mechanism of diffusion across the membrane. Thus, the systematic investigation of chemical structure-permeability relationships in the simple two compartment cell has given us the best conceptualization of how the skin functions as a barrier. As permeability coefficient data become more numerous, it should be possible to predict, from structural considerations alone, the relative ease by which chemicals will permeate skin. Such information is necessary to select the best topical candidate from a family of drugs and even to decide whether transdermal delivery is feasible for a given drug. The finite dose diffusion cell, on the other hand, is a product development tool. It promises little insight into the permeation mechanism per se, but at the same time it allows a researcher to acquire useful, formulation-directing data on the real and very complex formulations and systems used to administer drugs topically.

II. TECHNIQUES OF DATA REDUCTION

As suggested above, data on the two-compartment diffusion cell can be reduced to quantitative, characteristic mass transfer (permeability) coefficients if the experimental circumstances are properly adjusted. To a limited extent, the techniques of analysis developed for the two-compartment cell might also be applied to finite dose cell data. This would be possible, for instance, in some cases where the drug was only partially dissolved with the undissolved solid acting as a reservoir. However, with this latter cell one will, more usually, compare whole profiles rather than try to estimate, at best, very approximate permeability coefficients. This would be especially so when the vehicle is complex and the state of solubility of a drug within it is in question or when the vehicle undergoes significant compositional changes over the course of delivering a drug.

The most common manner of operation of a two-compartment diffusion cell involves the use of two-reservoir half-cells with fixed volumes. After placing a membrane in between, the reservoirs are filled with a fluid medium (often a physiologic, aqueous medium) and on one side of the membrane (donor) a chemical charge is introduced. This can be added to the phase before it is placed in the cell or as a concentrate after the compartment is filled with blank solvent. Typically, samples are drawn periodically from the other half-cell (receiver) and a plot of the amount accumulated as a function of time is made (Figure 1). Under circumstances where the concentration difference across the membrane is invariant or very nearly so, a steady state (or quasi-steady state) develops in the rate of build-up of mass in the receiver and, as long as there is no significant accumulation of mass in the membrane itself, the steady state rate is related to the mass transfer (permeability) coefficient by

$$\frac{dM}{dt} = AP\,(\Delta C) \tag{1}$$

where A is the area of the membrane through which the diffusion is taking place (the area of the opening of the half-cell), ΔC is the concentration different across the half-cells (usually nicely approximated by the donor cell concentration), and P is the mass transfer coefficient. Furthermore, since

$$\left(\frac{dM}{dt}\right) = V_r \left(\frac{dC}{dt}\right)_{ss} \tag{2}$$

the process can be followed as the changing concentration in the receiver half-cell and corrected to changing mass by introducing the volume of the receiver half-cell. This configuration also allows the estimation of the diffusional lag time via extrapolation of the steady state to the time axis. For a simple homogeneous membrane operating without influence of hydrodynamic layers, the lag time is related to the membrane diffusion coefficient of the permeant through

$$t_L = \frac{h^2}{6D} \tag{3}$$

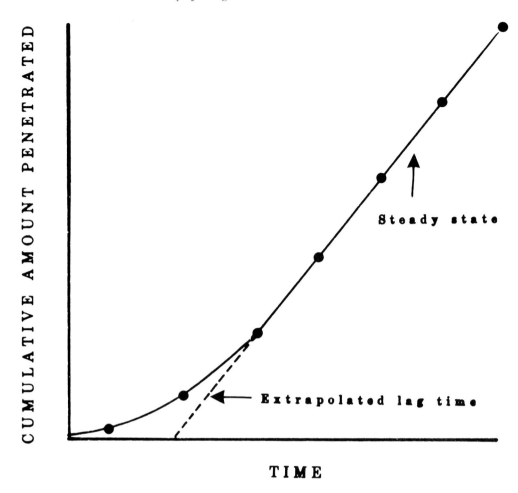

FIGURE 1.   A typical receiver accumulation profile for a two-compartment diffusion cell under conditions which yield a steady state or quasisteady state. The slope of the linear portion of the curve is the steady-state rate of diffusional transfer of matter. Extrapolation of this line to the time axis yields the diffusional lag time, which can be looked upon as the time it takes for the diffusion gradient to be fully expressed across the membrane.

where t_L is the lag time, h is the membrane thickness, and D is the diffusion coefficient (diffusivity). For complex membranes as the skin, one only obtains an apparent diffusivity from this extrapolation but even this has its uses in barrier characterization.

Another way the cell system can be configured is to use a standard reservoir half-cell for the donor compartment and a flow through half-cell for the receiver. The receiver is continuously and copiously rinsed to maintain zero concentration on this side. In this mode under usual circumstances, the rate of loss of material from the donor compartment becomes first order after the brief time needed to establish the membrane gradient (Figure 2) and thus, one can write

$$\frac{dC}{dt} = -kC \tag{4}$$

and therefore

$$\ell n \left(\frac{C_t}{C_o} \right) = kt \tag{5}$$

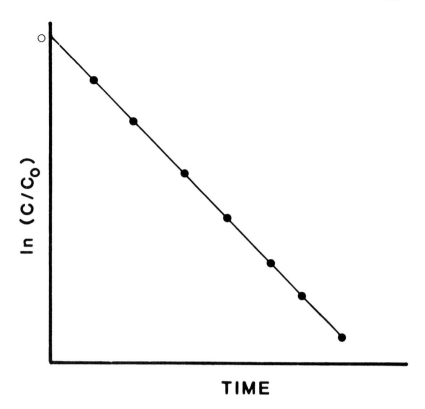

FIGURE 2.   This drawing illustrates an alternative way to follow the time course of diffusion of a substance across a membrane into a sink. In this case, the donor concentration is plotted semilogarithmically against time. The first order rate constant obtained is related to the permeability coefficient as expressed in Equation 6 in the text.

where C_t is the donor concentration at time t and C_o is the initial donor concentration. The first order rate constant, k, has the following relationship to the mass transfer (permeability) coefficient

$$k = \frac{P \cdot A}{V_d} \tag{6}$$

where A is the area and V_d is the donor half-cell volume. This particular approach is useful when the rate of skin permeation is relatively fast, as it tends to be for low molecular weight, hydrophobic chemicals, and it may be the only workable procedure when the solubility of the chemical involved is so low relative to the analytical method that quantitation of the small amounts of the drug which permeate while the permeation process is in a quasi-steady state by the first mentioned method is impossible. The latter condition arises with very hydrophobic chemicals if, as is usually done, the vehicle chosen is essentially water.

A third way to obtain the mass transfer coefficient (Figure 3) is by repetitive exchange of the donor phase and receiver phase to re-establish the initial conditions for both at fixed, identical time intervals. Here the data are recorded as the amount penetrated per interval (rather than cumulative amount) and a histogram as shown in the third illustration is prepared. When the amount per interval passing onto the receiver compartment is the same interval after interval and also equal to the amount depleted from the donor, one has approximated the conditions of a steady state and the mass transfer coefficient is found through

$$\frac{\Delta M}{\Delta t} \simeq \frac{dM}{dt} = AP(\Delta C) \tag{7}$$

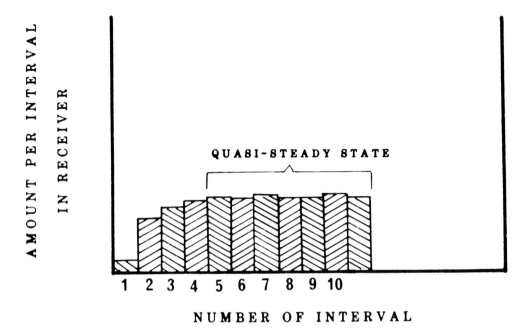

FIGURE 3.   A histogram of the accumulation of permeant in the receiver compartment of the two-compartment diffusion cell over a constant interval of time from the beginning of the diffusion process until a steady state or its very near approximation is reached. To use this technique of treating the data, one must exchange both donor and receiver cell contents with donor and receiver solutions of the original concentration at the beginning of each time interval. By this technique, errors introduced by heavy retention of the permeant substance in the membrane are forced to cancel one another and a close approximation of a true steady state is achieved.

where ΔM is the finite mass increment accumulated in the fixed, finite time interval, Δt. Here again, A is the membrane area and P is the mass transfer (permeability) coefficient. The term, ΔC, is now taken as the average difference or mid-interval difference in concentration across the diffusion cell during this interval. This is a relatively novel approach. It, too, works best when the permeation process is relatively rapid so that 20 to 25% of the material in the donor compartment at the beginning of a reasonable interval finds itself in the receiver at the end of the interval. One wants to check that the loss from the donor phase is exactly equal to the gain in the receiver phase when using this method. We have carefully tested the technique and find it useful in those instances where the membrane retains a significant amount of the diffusing substance, a condition which obviates the use of the other two techniques of data reduction. However, the first technique can always be applied if trouble is taken to force true steady-state conditions. In this case, the quantity of material retained in the membrane is invariant once the true steady state is reached and the permeability coefficient is accurately reflected in the flux. The finite interval technique might be the best technique for hydrophobic drugs as these tend to accumulate to a significant extent in the skin.

III. IN VITRO STRATEGIES

At this point it seems worthwhile to briefly indicate something of the techniques and physicochemical probes related to permeability one can use to define the operational characteristics of a complex membrane barrier as the skin. First, one must recognize that all biological membranes are heterogeneous and composed of distinct macroscopic phases and the passive diffusive current across such complex membranes is dependent on the organization and sequencing of all encountered phases in the permeation process. Permeation is also dependent on the physicochemical natures of the phases such as their densities and viscosities, both of which affect rates of diffusive movement of matter, and on the relative physico-chemical interactions between the permeant and the respective phases as reflected in solubilities and partition coefficients.

All phases in a membrane may be characterized in terms of a diffusional resistance. Furthermore, a membrane may be regarded as making a circuit between two external phases (between the donor and receptor compartments of a diffusion cell or between the vehicle and the systemic circulation). The mass current will depend upon the nature and organization of the circuitry or on the phase resistances and their arrangement. Phases to be encountered can be arranged in series as the distinct layers of the epidermis are arranged or, in parallel, as the appendages are placed relative to the stratum corneum or, they may appear as some form of dispersion in the diffusional field. When arranged in series, the diffusional flux for a given chemical potential drop across the membrane is determined by the sum of the resistances of the strata. Mathematically, the amount penetrating the membrane as a function of time, dM/dt, in the steady state in an uncomplicated series case can be represented by

$$\left(\frac{dM}{dt}\right) = A \cdot \left[\frac{1}{R_1 + R_2 + \dots R_n}\right] \cdot \Delta C \tag{8}$$

where A and ΔC have the meanings defined in Equation 1 and the term

$$\frac{1}{R_1 + R_2 + \dots R_n}$$

is the permeability coefficient, P, for this particular case. It will be noted that Equation 8 is of the same form as Equation 1 except that the mass transfer parameter is given a more detailed definition. Indeed, Equation 1 is general and holds regardless of membrane composition and permeation mechanism. Membrane characterization, therefore, is seen to be a matter of appropriately representing P in terms of series, parallel, and inclusion phase resistances.

When phases are aligned in parallel such that there can be independent currents through each, the total steady-state flux is simply the sum of the individual fluxes of the parallel pathways adjusted for their fractional membrane areas, f_i. For the uncomplicated case of multiple parallel pathways

$$\left(\frac{dM}{dt}\right) = A \cdot [f_1 P_1 + f_2 P_2 + \dots f_n P_n] \cdot \Delta C \tag{9}$$

where the term $[f_1 P_1 + f_2 P_2 + \dots f_n P_n]$ now defines the overall permeability coefficient, P. The individual permeability coefficient for an isolated phase (whether series or parallel or otherwise) is the reciprocal of the diffusional resistance of that phase or, according to Flynn, Yalkowsky, and Roseman[1]

$$P_i = \frac{1}{R_i} \tag{10}$$

Equation 9 can now be rewritten in the form

$$\left(\frac{dM}{dt}\right) = A \cdot \left[\frac{f_1}{R_1} + \frac{f_2}{R_2} + \dots + \frac{f_n}{R_n}\right] \cdot \Delta C \tag{11}$$

It can be seen, then, that the permeability coefficient for phases in series is the reciprocal of the summed resistances while for phases in parallel it is the sum of area-adjusted reciprocals of the resistances. The very complex circuitries of real membranes can often be broken down into manageable components in this fashion.

In exact modeling, the distortions of flow lines resulting from the arrangements of phases within phases also have to be considered but most biological membranes cannot be dealt with at this level of detail, the uncertainties as to composition, geometry, density of packing, etc. of the particles are so great. Rather and as a practical matter, flowline distortions which relate to inclusion bodies are taken up in permeability coefficients of the pathway in which the dispersed matter is formed and one works with effective, composite permeability parameters.

The diffusional resistance of a phase can be explicitly defined in terms of the thickness of the phase in question, h; the permeant diffusion coefficient (diffusivity) in the phase, D, which relates to molecular mobility; and the relative conduit capacity of the phase which is directly related to the equilibrium distribution of the permeant between that membrane phase and the principle external phase as expressed in the partition coefficient, K. The simple mathematical definition is

$$R_i = \frac{h_i}{D_i K_i} \tag{12}$$

It now becomes a straightforward matter to recast Equations 8 and 9 in terms of the thicknesses, diffusivities, and partition coefficients of the respective phases. Membrane characterization then becomes a matter of systematically and selectively altering the resistance determining parameters by membrane preparation or treatment, by choice of permeants or by manipulation of the vehicle. Such physicochemical maneuvering alters the relative resistances of various phases and the patterns of permeability which develop say much about the nature of the rate controlling phase or phases.

Included among the tools at ones disposal to predictably and selectively alter the rate-controlling parameters are

1.   The use of homologs, as these have systematically changing partition coefficients
2.   The choice of permeants of different sizes to deliberately alter diffusivity
3.   The variation of membrane or phase thickness by several means
4.   pH effects
5.   The inhibition of membrane enzymes
6.   The treatment of membranes with heat and solvents and other chemicals which selectively alter critical phase properties

Each of these factors will be examined in the following section and some of the characteristics of each factor which make it useful for manipulating and interpreting barrier attributes of the skin will be highlighted.

A. Homolog Partitioning Effects

Partitioning is a most critical factor governing the relative rates of permeation of analogs and homologs through lipophilic membranes. The following theoretical discussion of solution phase behavior and its relationship to partitioning for a given compound and between compounds thus sets the stage for further conceptual development of diffusional processes.

When a molecule is changed by the addition of functional groups as in the making of derivatives and analogs of drugs, the activity coefficients of the formed compounds in phases of the skin as well as in simple solvents selected for partitioning are altered. Each added moiety causes fixed changes in distribution coefficients between each pair of encountered phases and thus fixed changes in the free energies of transfer related thereto. Distinct functional group-free energies of transfer are associated with each added functional moiety and free energies for transfer are usually considered constant and additive for successive incremental additions of the same functional group at comparable positions to a parent molecule when the partitioning is between a set pair of immiscible solvents. The logarithm of the increase or decrease in partitioning as measured in the ratio of two partition coefficients will be constant with each like functional group added, giving a linear relationship between the logarithm of the partition coefficient and the number of like functional groups added. Thus, for a homologous series, where methylene units are added in linear chains, the free energy of transfer between immiscible phases, one of which is usually considered aqueous, increases linearly with extension of the alkyl chain. It follows that a plot of the logarithm of the partition coefficients of alkyl homologs against their alkyl chainlength will be linear with a slope of

$$\pi_{CH_2} = \frac{d(\log K)}{dn} \tag{13}$$

While π can represent the contribution to partitioning of any substituent, its use in membrane studies has generally been limited to the methylene unit.

The changes in the activity coefficient in each of the phases is reflected in π as the alkyl chain is varied and thus, in principle, it takes a different value for a given homologous series partitioning between different immiscible "oils" and water. Such is generally observed and the π constant reportedly varies[2] from about 0.3 to 0.6. It might be noted at this point that partitioning relationships as these are spoken of as extrathermodynamic. This term arises from the fact that there is no provision in classical thermodynamics for comparison of activities between different chemical species. Rather, the reference state is defined for each chemical as a unique species and in standard approaches each species is compared to its own reference state. Thus, when comparisons in free energies between different molecular species are drawn, as they essentially are in computing substituent-free energies of partitioning, thermodynamics slips outside its classical bounds.

The relationships between partitioning and the permeability of the membrane to homologs measured from external aqueous media over certain regions of polarity are well established. For instance, Ho et al.[3] found a correlation between partitioning into and permeability of the buccal membrane to the alkanoic acids. Scheuplein[4] found that alkanol permeation of human skin paralleled partitioning in the stratum corneum. Durrheim et al.[5] found that, for the homologous n-alkanols, permeability coefficients through hairless mouse skin paralleled partition coefficients, at least at intermediate chainlengths. Flynn and Yalkowsky[6] found that, for the homologous n-alkyl p-amino benzoates, permeability coefficients also paralleled partitioning in silicone rubber membranes over an extended range of esters. However, and importantly, in all of the instances cited, there is evidence at long alkyl chain length of a change in rate-determining mechanism and a loss of *direct* partitioning sensitivity of the mass transfer processes. This is attributable to the coming into play of an aqueous resistance in series with that of the membrane. Minimally hydrodynamic layers are involved and tissues as the skin also have watery phases in series with their lipid regimes.

To this point the discussion has essentially dealt with partitioning under circumstances where there are but two solvent phases. However, all biological membranes and even some synthetic membranes are polyphasic and equilibrium distribution into such complex media must be characterized in terms of each participating region. In the biological case, three general types of phases can be hypothesized in terms of their relative polarities. First, there are strictly aqueous regions such as the bulk of the cytoplasm and the extracellular water.

Second, there are semipolar regions of which certain protein masses may be representative. Third, there are hydrophobic regions which are accumulations of lipids and other truly nonpolar substances such as found in the cell membranes and certain cellular organelles. These regions are similar to those suggested by Higuchi and Davis[7] for their structure/activity model for multiphasic systems. If we let the subscript, AQ, stand for the aqueous regions; HB, stand for the hydrophobic regions, and SP stand for the proteinaceous regions, then at equilibrium, the total amount of drug in the membrane is equal to the sum of the amounts in each of the separate regions of the membrane. That is

$$M_m = M_{AQ} + M_{SP} + M_{HB} \tag{14}$$

The concentration of drug in the aqueous solution bathing the membrane is C_w. The apparent partition coefficient, K_{app} is equal to the ratio of the concentration of the drug in the membrane to that in the aqueous phase:

$$K_{app} = \frac{C_m}{C_w} \tag{15}$$

C_m may be represented as the amount in the membrane divided by the volume of the membrane:

$$C_m = \frac{M_m}{V_m} = \frac{M_{AQ} + M_{SP} + M_{HB}}{V_m} \tag{16}$$

It is readily seen that the total amount in the membrane can also be represented as:

$$M_m = C_w (K_{AQ}V_{AQ} + K_{SP}V_{SP} + K_{HB}V_{HB}) \tag{17}$$

where

$$K_i = \frac{C_i}{C_w} \tag{18}$$

that is, each region is in partitioning equilibrium with the external bathing solution. Therefore,

$$K_{app} = \frac{C_w \, \Sigma \, K_i V_i / V_m}{C_w} = \frac{\Sigma \, K_i V_i}{V_m} \tag{19}$$

Individual K_is may vary depending on the region into which the compounds partition and on the nature of the compounds themselves, but the overall distribution coefficient, K_{app}, may or may not reflect these changes depending on the magnitudes of all $K_i V_i$.

This equation points out how important it is to consider the volume of the region into which the drug is partitioned as well as the microscopic partition coefficient under circumstances where membrane is polyphasic. Since the permeability coefficient, P, may be directly proportional to K_{app} and is, at least, a function of the microscopic partition coefficients for the individual phases, then permeability coefficients for a series may depend on how the various K_i change with extension of the alkyl chain. Clearly they may also depend on the relative magnitudes of the volumes of the various phases in the membrane. Where the membrane is polyphasic in nature, π may not be a relatively constant value, and may even change with each successive addition of a methylene group. If we assume that the membrane is only biphasic in nature, and that the two phases are aqueous and hydrophobic in nature, then we have two potential partitioning dependencies, K_{AQ}, and K_{HB} and also two phase volumes, V_{AQ} and V_{HB}. Therefore,

$$K_{app} = \frac{K_{AQ} \, V_{AQ} + K_{HB} \, V_{HB}}{V_m} \tag{20}$$

These partitioning relationships are experimentally well established for skin tissue. For instance, Scheuplein has demonstrated a biphasic relationship for partitioning in hydrated human stratum corneum.[8] Durrheim et al.[5] have shown the same to be true for the skin of the hairless mouse, K_{app} being unchanged up to butanol, where it begins an exponential increase with further extension of the alkyl chain. The close correlation between equilibrium partition coefficients and permeability coefficients for the alkanols permeating human skin and hairless mouse skin suggests that the regions of the skin (stratum corneum) into which they are partitioning and the regions governing the permeation process may be the same. This need not be generally true. Depending on the magnitude of the individual K_i and on the microscopic volumes and arrangements of the phases of the membrane, points of transition in K_{app} may not coincide with fundamental, mechanistically important transitions in barrier behavior.

All of the above observations relating the membrane permeability coefficients of homologs to their membrane/water partition coefficients are the direct consequence of the simple resistance equation for the ith phase of a membrane. Of utmost importance when lipids are the medium of transport, phase resistances decrease as partition coefficients increase, which means that permeability (the reciprocal of resistance) grows exponentially with chain length. Thus, the existence of an exponential trend in permeability coefficients is sufficient evidence to ascribe lipid properties to a membrane. It should be pointed out that there may not be perfect agreement in the slopes of equilibrium partitioning and permeability patterns due to concurrent but slight decreases in diffusivity as molecular volume is increased. However, in most instances involving homologs such shifts in diffusivity as do occur are inconsequential. It follows then that the steepness of the slope of a plot of the logarithm of the permeability coefficient vs. alkyl chain length can itself be informative as long as diffusivities are essentially invariant. This is so because the activity coefficient change in the lipid phase,

$$\frac{d \log \gamma_{HB}}{dn} \tag{21}$$

is sensitive to the polarity of the phase for a given homologous series. The more nonpolar a phase, the more negative this quantity tends to be and thus the greater is the π-value. Very steep slopes on homolog permeability plots signal a very nonpolar lipid phase while shallow slopes suggest that the diffusional medium tends toward the semipolar side. For a given homologous series, the π value for a strictly apolar phase can be obtained using synthetic membranes made of materials such as silicone rubber, or, failing this, can be approximated from actual distribution coefficients between apolar solvents and water.

In contrast, when under the same conditions as described above, the permeability coefficients of the members of a homologous series applied in aqueous media are invariant, one has necessary and sufficient information to describe the operative phase of the membrane as an aqueous phase. In the resistance equation, (Equation 12) the thickness h_i, is constant unless deliberately manipulated and, again, D_i does not vary greatly. Thus an invariant P_i means that $1/K_i$ or, more explicitly, K_i itself is invariant. This will only occur when the phase of the membrane supporting most of the diffusional current is physicochemically essentially the same as water such that $K_i \sim 1.0$. On this basis "aqueous pore pathways" have been postulated for a number of biological membranes and, indeed, seem to also exist within the stratum corneum.[9] When there is a change in partitioning dependency of permeability there is necessarily a change in the rate-controlling mechanism for diffusion. Such observations are enormously significant clues to the barrier mechanisms of complex membranes.

B. Structure/Diffusivity Relationships

Equation 3 has given the relationship between the duration of the nonstationary state (lag time) and diffusivity for a simple isotropic membrane. It should be noted that diffusivity also exerts a direct influence on steady-state fluxes and permeability coefficients derived therefrom as seen in the general resistance equation (Equation 12). It follows that differences in diffusivity brought about through judicious selection of permeants can exert influence on permeability patterns which are mechanistically interpretive. Because diffusivities decrease rapidly as the radius of a permeant approaches the radius of the pore it is passing through, molecular size effects (diffusivity effects) have particularly been used to probe pore sizes of biologic membranes such as in the gastrointestinal tract. Little use of such techniques has been made with the skin, however, though this could be conceptually rewarding as pointed out below.

The diffusivity of a drug molecule in a medium is dependent on the properties and the degree of interaction between the diffusant and the medium. As suggested, it can be highly sensitive to pore size. The effect of structural modification on diffusivity is the alteration of frictional resistance that a diffusant experiences in moving through a medium. Diffusivities in liquid media in general tend to decrease with an increase in molecular volume according to[1]

$$D \propto V^{-1/3}$$

Thus, molecular diffusivity in liquid is expected to vary only slightly with increased molecular size. On the other hand, in more structured media such as semicrystalline polymer matrices, diffusivities of homologs tend to exhibit exaggerated molecular size dependencies.[10] Diffusion through molecularly porous living cells, such as Chara cells,[11] is also found to be highly sensitive to molecular size, the overall effect approaching that seen in some rigid polymers.[10]

The effect of adsorptive phenomena on permeability as discussed by Flynn and Roseman[12] has possible significance to the behavior of skin, or more specifically stratum corneum, as a membrane. If keratin can be considered a dispersed phase in the skin that is capable of adsorbing or binding a permeant, then lag times may be lengthened by the initial removal of an amount of permeant from the diffusional stream. Diffusivities calculated in the usual fashion from the Daynes and Barrer lag time relationship (Equation 22) are much smaller than the true diffusivity to the extent this occurs. Unusually small diffusivities may especially be seen with polar, polyfunctional permeants as such molecules have many possible points of attachment to the immobilized proteins of the skin.

The above feature of lag times suggests that lag times per se may indicate something of the mechanism of barrier resistance. For instance, where binding to an internal phase is irreversible, lag times have a concentration dependency and their lengthening as concentration is decreased is unequivocal proof of such sorption. Such behavior also warns that Daynes and Barrer's diffusivity calculations will be in error and that an alternative approach to estimating diffusivities must be found. Obviously, where lag times are uncomplicated, they provide reasonable estimates of effective diffusivities. Finally, lag time relationships change as boundary layer control of permeabilities is attained in the course of ascending a homologous series and an exponentially increasing lag time with increasing alkyl chain length is another sign of a transition of rate controlling phases from lipid strata to aqueous strata.[6]

C. Changing Membrane or Phase Thickness

For a homogeneous membrane, h is simply the thickness of the membrane. For a heterogeneous membrane, the effective thickness, H, can be greater than the true membrane width if the permeant must follow a tortuous route through the membrane. To adjust membrane thickness to account for deviations in the path that a molecule must take in crossing the membrane, the actual thickness of the membrane is related to the effective thickness through a factor called the tortuosity, τ. H is equal to τh and the simple Daynes and Barrer lag time expression becomes

$$t_L = \frac{h^2\tau^2}{6D} = \frac{H^2}{6D} \tag{22}$$

This expression is applicable to a heterogeneous membrane with a nonabsorbing internally tortuous phase. The intercellular path through the stratum corneum proposed by some[13,14] is highly tortuous and long lag times are to be expected.

The resistance of a phase is directly proportional to the thickness of the phase. In the casting of synthetic membranes, thickness and, thus, membrane resistance are generally quite easily manipulated. It is possible to accentuate the influences of boundary layers by systematically thinning the membrane.[15] Changing the thickness of biological membranes is generally more difficult if not impossible to do. Where skin is involved, sections can be forcibly cut into different thicknesses by varying the setting of a dermatome. Presently no dermatome is capable of shaving the thin stratum corneum into thin sections. However, the stratum corneum is a laminated structure and to a degree layered structure can be thinned and even removed by tape stripping. This procedure has been used by many investigators to systematically alter the role that the stratum corneum plays in percutaneous absorption.[16-17]

D. Hydrodynamic Boundary Layers and Stirring Effects

A situation often encountered in permeation experiments is the slowing of transport by stagnant layers of water or bathing media which are generated at the surface of a membrane under study. For long-chain-length homologs, the flux of a compound across the membrane may be controlled by the rate of diffusion of the compound across the hydrodynamic barrier. Hydrodynamic boundary layers exist at a fluid-solid interface any time a fluid and solid are moving at different velocities with respect to each other and there is a "viscous drag" at the interface. In the diffusion cell, the fluid media are stirred and the membrane in between is stationary and so-called "unstirred layers" are generated at each interface of the membrane. These represent liquid regions where mixing by forced convection is so limited that diffusive events become more important than mixing itself. Thus, the boundary layers are essentially crossed by passive diffusion or natural convection. These represent sources of diffusional resistance in series with the resistance of the membrane. As the facility of crossing the membrane phase is increased, as it is by making the membrane very thin or by increasing the membrane/water partition coefficient, aqueous boundary layers play an increasingly important role in mass transfer and can become rate determining in the extremes of reduction of the resistance of the membrane.[6,15] Also, by increasing or decreasing the stirring rate, the thickness of this stagnant barrier may also be altered to allow for slightly altered rates of movement across the membrane-boundary layer composite barrier.[15] Techniques such as varying the stirring rate are used to show if and to what extent the boundary layers are involved in the mass transfer kinetics.

E. Inhibition of Membrane Binding

A second permeant capable of altering adsorption and binding processes in the membrane (which may be associated with membrane metabolism) will change the time course of a diffusional experiment in an interpretable way. Lag times are shortened and it is at least theoretically possible to infer the lag time for the sorptionless case and thereby estimate the actual diffusivity.

F. Membrane Sectioning Techniques

Often it is possible to separate membranes into layers either mechanically or chemically. For example, the epidermis of human skin can be mechanically separated from the dermis by treatment with water at 60°C for 30 sec to 1 min and the stratum corneum may be isolated by enzymatic digestion of the living epidermal layers by trypsin. The whole epidermis may also be loosened and isolated by prolonged soaking in water at 37°C. The epidermis may then be removed as a contiguous sheet by careful separation from the dermis. These techniques allow one to characterize the diffusional resistances of specific layers of the skin and therefore to assign the rate control of the intact skin to one or more of its principal strata. Such techniques were particularly well applied by Scheuplein[4] and by Flynn et al.[17] to the permeability of human and mouse skin membranes, respectively.

G. Chemical and Thermal Treatment of Membranes

By treating the epidermis with a strong lipid solvent or a combination of solvents such as methanol and chloroform, it is possible to remove the lipids from the membrane selectively, a subject treated in detail in the chapter on skin condition and function. Comparison of the permeation rates before and after treatment has been used to decipher the role lipids play in controlling skin permeation. Similarly, heat and certain chemicals can be used to selectively denature or alter phases of complex biological membranes and probe the role of proteins within the barrier.

In our labs, we have found that heating skin above 80°C leads to a marked increase in permeability which is apparently attributable to denaturation of keratin.[18] Phenol, a known protein denaturant, has the same ability at high concentrations as seen with work on human epidermal membranes[19] and mouse skin.[20] Such techniques serve to illustrate the importance of the organization of the protein (keratin) phase to the barrier functioning of the stratum corneum.

IV. SUMMARY

The above discussion shows structure/permeability behaviors reveal a great deal about the functionality of membranes. Moreover, when the membrane can be broken down into its constituent strata, much can be learned of the functioning of its individual phases. Selective chemical and other membrane treatments are also showing us the relative importance of distinct regions which form critical parts of the skin barrier. Overall, these techniques applied to the skin show the stratum corneum to have a significant lipophilic character but also reveal that very polar substances and even ions permeate at measurable rates. There must be several pathways, one of which supports the limited flux of lipid insoluble substances. Moreover, we have learned that the unique organization of the proteins of the healthy horny layer is critical to its high diffusional resistance to most substances. The same is true for its intercellular lipid. These techniques also suggest that the living epidermis and dermis offer no more than a nominal aqueous resistance to the diffusion of most substances. Thus, once the horny layer is removed or destroyed, absorption of all substances not readily passing through intact stratum corneum with facility is made facile. All of this is giving us a deeper appreciation of the barrier of the skin and inching us closer to the time when absorption rates through skin can be estimated *a priori*.

REFERENCES

1. **Flynn, G. L., Yalkowsky, S. H., and Roseman, T. J.,** Mass transport phenomena and models: theoretical aspects, *J. Pharm. Sci.,* 63, 479, 1975.
2. **Davis, S. S., Higuchi, T., and Rytting, J. H.,** Determination of thermodynamics of functional groups in solutions of drug moelcules, *Advances in Pharmaceutical Sciences,* Vol. 4, Bean, H. S., Beckett, A. H., and Carless, J. E., Eds., Academic Press, New York, 1974, 73.
3. **Ho, N. F., Park, J. Y., Morosowich, W., and Higuchi, W. I.,** Physical model approach to the design of drugs with improced intestinal absorption, *Design of Biopharmaceutical Properties Through Prodrugs and Analogs,* E. B. Roche, Ed., American Pharmaceutical Association, Academy of Pharmaceutical Sciences, Washington, D.C., 1977, 136.
4. **Scheuplein, R.,** Skin permeation, *The Physiology and Pathophysiology of the Skin,* Jarrett, A., Ed., Academic Press, New York, 1975, 1693.
5. **Durrheim, H. H., Flynn, G. L., Higuchi, W. I., and Behl, C. R.,** Permeation of hairless mouse skin. I. Experimental methods and comparison with human epidermal permeation by alkanols, *J. Pharm. Sci.,* 69, 781, 1980.
6. **Flynn, G. L. and Yalkowsky, S. H.,** Correlation and prediction of mass transport across membranes. I. Influence of alkyl chain length on the flux determining properties of barrier and diffusant, *J. Pharm. Sci.,* 61, 838, 1972.
7. **Higuchi, T. and Davis, S. S.,** Thermodynamic analysis of structure-activity relationships of drugs: prediction of optimal structure, *J. Pharm. Sci.,* 59, 1376, 1970.
8. **Scheuplein, R. J.,** Mechanism of percutaneous adsorption. I. Routes of penetration and the influence of solubility, *J. Invest. Dermatol.,* 45, 334, 1965.
9. **Scheuplein, R. J. and Blank, I. H.,** Permeability of the skin, *Physiol. Rev.,* 51, 702, 1971.
10. **Kumins, C. A. and Kovei, T. K.,** Free volume and other theories, in *Diffusion in Polymers,* Crank, J. and Park, G. S., Eds., Academic Press, New York, 1968, 107.
11. **Collander, R. and Barlund, H.,** Permeabilitats-studien an Chara ceratophylla, *Acta Bot. Fenn.,* 2, 1, 1933.
12. **Flynn, G. L. and Roseman, T. J.,** Membrane diffusion. II. Influence of physical absorption on molecular flux through heterogeneous dimethylpolysiloxane barriers, *J. Pharm. Sci.,* 60, 1788, 1971.
13. **Elias, P. M.,** Lipids and the epidermal barrier, *Arch. Dermatol. Res.,* 270, 95, 1981.
14. **Blank, I. H. and Scheuplein, R. J.,** The epidermal barrier, in *Progress in the Biological Sciences in Relation to Dermatology,* Vol. 2, Rook, A. and Champion, R. H., Eds., Cambridge University Press, London, 1965, 245.
15. **Flynn, G. L., French, A. B., Ho, N. F. H., Higuchi, W. I., Ostafin, E. A., Warbasse, L. H., Amidon, G. E., and Williams, E.,** Some hydrodynamic boundary layer influences on mass transfer coefficients, *J. Membr. Sci.,* 19, 289, 1984.
16. **Blank, I. H.,** Further observation on factors which influence the water content of the stratum corneum, *J. Invest. Dermatol.,* 21, 259, 1953.
17. **Flynn, G. L., Durrheim, H. H., and Higuchi, W. I.,** Permeation of hairless mouse skin. II. Membrane sectioning techniques and influences on alkanol permeabilities, *J. Pharm. Sci.,* 70, 52, 1981.
18. **Flynn, G. L., Behl, C. R., Walters, K. A., Gatmaitan, O. G., Willkowsky, A., Kurihara, T., Ho, N. F. H., Higuchi, W. I., and Pierson, C. L.,** Permeability of thermally damaged skin. III. Influence of scalding temperature on mass transfer of water and *n*-alkanols across hairless mouse skin, *Burns,* 8, 47, 1981.
19. **Roberts, M. S., Anderson, R. A., and Swarbrick, J.,** Permeability of Human epidermis to phenolic compounds, *J. Pharm. Pharmacol.,* 29, 677, 1977.
20. **Behl, C. R., Linn, E. E., Flynn, G. L., Pierson, C. L., Higuchi, W. I., and Ho, N. F. H.,** Permeation of skin and eschar by antiseptics. I. Baseline studies with phenol, *J. Pharm. Sci.,* 72, 391, 1983.

Chapter 5

ANIMAL MODELS FOR TRANSDERMAL DELIVERY

Ronald C. Wester and Howard I. Maibach

TABLE OF CONTENTS

I. INTRODUCTION

The ideal way to determine the transdermal delivery potential of a compound in man is to do the actual study in man. Mechanisms and parameters of transdermal delivery elucidated in vivo with human skin are most relevant to the clinical situation. However, the cost and complexity of studies in vivo in man are immense. Therefore, preclinical studies are needed to determine the potential toxicity and efficacy/bioavailability before clinical studies are undertaken. This involves the use of animals, either in vivo or the use of animal skin, in vitro. The following is a discussion of the validity of animal models for percutaneous absorption and transdermal delivery.

A. Comparative In Vivo Studies

The basic data for in vivo human percutaneous absorption, to which animal models are compared, were obtained from Feldmann and Maibach.[1-3] In these clinical studies, a specific concentration of radioactive compound (4 $\mu g/cm^2$) was applied to a specific anatomical site (ventral forearm); the area was not occluded and subjects were requested not to wash the area for 24 hr. The radioactive compounds were applied to the skin in an acetone solution and the acetone quickly evaporated with a gentle stream of air. Urine was collected for 5 days and assayed for radioactivity. A tracer dose was also given parenterally, and the percent radioactivity in the urine following parenteral administration was used to correct for compound which might be excreted by some other route and for a compound which might be retained within the body.

Bartek et al.[4] undertook a comparative study of percutaneous absorption in rats, rabbits, miniature swine, and man. Methodology in the animals was similar to that in man except that in animals the compounds were applied to the skin of the back and the site of application was shaved. Radioactive compounds were applied to the skin in the same manner that had been used in man. A nonoccluding device was used to keep the animal from removing the applied compound. This study showed rabbit skin to be the most permeable to topically applied compounds, followed closely by rat skin. In contrast, it appears that the permeability of the skin of the miniature swine is closer to that of human skin (Table 1). Clearly, percutaneous absorption in the rabbit and rat would not be predictive of that in man. It is not known if the subtle differences seen between pig and human skin were due to methodology (site of application, shaving) or the skin itself. However, generally the pig appears to be a good predictor of percutaneous absorption in man.

Bartek and LaBudde[5] also studied the percutaneous absorption of pesticides in the rabbit, pig, and squirrel monkey, and compared the results with the absorption obtained in man. The methodology used was the same as their previous studies. The compounds were also applied to the back of the squirrel monkey. The results were compared to man where the site of application was the ventral forearm. It appears that the in vivo percutaneous absorption of pesticides in the rabbit was again much greater than in man, whereas penetration in the pig and squirrel monkey was closer to that of man (Table 2).

Several comparisons of percutaneous absorption in the rhesus monkey and in man were made by Wester and Maibach.[6-10] Methodology and the site of application (ventral forearm) were the same for both species. The site of application was lightly clipper-shaved in the monkey. A direct comparison of unshaven and lightly clipper-shaved skin showed no difference in absorption.[6] Table 3 summarizes the results of these studies. The in vivo percutaneous absorption of hydrocortisone, testosterone, and benzoic acid was similar for the rhesus monkey and man. Also, the dose response was similar in the two species.

Andersen et al.[11] determined the percutaneous absorption of hydrocortisone, testosterone, and benzoic acid in the guinea pig and compared the results to man. A concentration of 4 $\mu g/cm^2$ of the ^{14}C-labeled compound was applied to the shaved backs of the animals and

Table 1
IN VIVO PERCUTANEOUS
ABSORPTION OF SEVERAL
COMPOUNDS BY RAT, RABBIT, PIG,
AND MAN

Chemical	Dose absorbed (%)			
	Rat	**Rabbit**	**Pig**	**Man**
Haloprogin	95.8	113.0	19.7	11.0
Acetylcysteine	3.5	2.0	6.0	2.4
Cortisone	24.7	30.3	4.1	3.4
Caffeine	53.1	69.2	32.4	47.6
Butter yellow	48.2	100.0	41.9	21.6
Testosterone	47.4	69.6	29.4	13.2

From Bartek et al., *J. Invest. Dermatol.*, 58, 114, 1972.
With permission.

Table 2
IN VIVO PERCUTANEOUS
ABSORPTION OF SEVERAL
PESTICIDES BY RABBIT, PIG,
SQUIRREL MONKEY, AND MAN

Chemical	Dose absorbed (%)			
	Rabbit	**Pig**	**Monkey**	**Man**
DDT	46.3	43.4	1.5	10.4
Lindane	51.2	37.6	16.0	9.3
Parathion	97.5	14.5	30.3	9.7
Malathion	64.6	15.5	19.3	8.2

From Bartek, M. J. and La Budde, J. A., *Animal Models in Dermatology: Relevance to Human Dermatopharmacology and Dermatotoxicology*, Churchill Livingston, London, 1975, 103. With permission.

percutaneous absorption determined from urinary and fecal excretion. Absorption of hydrocortisone and benzoic acid was similar to published human absorption data. However, testosterone was absorbed to a greater extent in guinea pigs than in man. The absorption value for testosterone in the guinea pig was closer to man if the radioactivity excretion in urine and feces were measured, rather than just the radioactivity excretion in urine alone. If a large proportion of the radioactivity is excreted in the feces, a more accurate estimate of the percutaneous absorption can be obtained by determining the radioactivity excretion in both urine and feces.[12]

Hunziker et al.[13] studied the percutaneous absorption of ^{14}C-labeled benzoic acid, progesterone, and testosterone in the Mexican hairless dog, and compared the absorption with that obtained in man. Total absorption and maximum absorption rates were greater in man than in the hairless dog. Surface counting experiments showed that benzoic acid and progesterone persisted on the dog skin far longer than on human skin.

In several of the preceding studies, the percutaneous absorption of testosterone was determined. In these studies, the same topical concentration, 4 µg/cm², was used. Additionally, the same method of analysis, determination of urinary ^{14}C-excretion, was used. Table 4

Table 3
IN VIVO PERCUTANEOUS
ABSORPTION OF INCREASED
TOPICAL DOSES OF SEVERAL
COMPOUNDS IN THE RHESUS
MONKEY AND MAN

Chemical	Dose (μg/cm^2)	Dose absorbed (%) Rhesus	Man
Hydrocortisone	4	2.9	1.9
	40	2.1	0.6
Benzoic acid	4	59.2	42.6
	40	33.6	25.7
	2000	17.4	14.4
Testosterone	4	18.4	13.2
	40	6.7	8.8[a]
	250	2.9	
	400	2.2	2.8
	1600	2.9	
	4000	1.4	

[a]   30 μg/cm^2

From Wester, R. C. and Noonan, P. K., *Int. J. Pharm.*, 7, 99, 1980. With permission.

Table 4
COMPARATIVE IN VIVO
PERCUTANEOUS
ABSORPTION OF
TESTOSTERONE IN
SEVERAL SPECIES

Species	Dose absorbed (%)
Rat	47.4
Rabbit	69.6
Guinea pig	34.9
Pig	29.4
Rhesus monkey	18.4
Man	13.2

From Wester, R. C. and Noonan, P. K., *Int. J. Pharm.*, 7, 99, 1980. With permission.

summarizes the results. Absorption of testosterone in the rat, rabbit, and guinea pig was high compared to man. Absorption in the pig was approximately twice that in man, and that in the rhesus monkey was closest to man. However, it must be remembered that even when the method and applied dose were the same, there were other differences besides species. The site of application in the rat, rabbit, guinea pig, and pig was the back, whereas in the rhesus monkey and man the site of application was the ventral forearm. Percutaneous absorption of testosterone in the rhesus monkey and man has been shown to vary with the site of application.[14,15] What proportions of the variation in the above comparison are due to species and due to the site of application is not known. However, it points out that when a difference is found, it could be a sum of the many variables in the study.

Table 5
IN VIVO TOPICAL BIOAVAILABILITY OF HAIR DYES

Species	Applied dose absorbed (%)		
	Resorcinol	2-Nitro-PPD	4-Amino-2-nitrophenol
Guinea pig	0.065	0.111	0.694
Monkey	0.016	0.508	—
Man	0.071	0.127	0.236

Table 6
EFFECT OF RUBBING CREAM ON DERMAL ABSORPTION OF CORTISONE: IN VIVO COMPARISON OF RHESUS MONKEY AND GUINEA PIG TO MAN

Specie	Percent cortisone dose absorbed (± SD)	
	Rub	Spread
Man	—	3.4 ± 1.6[a]
Rhesus monkey	6.2 ± 2.7	5.3 ± 3.3[b]
Guinea pig	20.0 ± 3.7	20.1 ± 4.3[b]

[a] Acetone vehicle.
[b] Cream vehicle.

From Feldmann, R. J. and Maibach, H. I., *J. Invest. Dermatol.*, 52, 89, 1969. With permission.

Table 5 gives the topical bioavailability of hair dyes in guinea pig, rhesus monkey, and man. The percent applied dose absorbed for the three hair dyes (resorcinol, 2-nitro-PPD, 4-amino-2-nitrophenol) was similar for each species, suggesting that the efficiency of absorption (percent) was the same. Obviously, the scalp area of man is larger than the scalp area of the monkey. Thus, more mass (microgram) would enter the human body than the monkey's body. However, for efficiency of absorption, the monkey and guinea pig appear to be predictive animal models for these hair dyes.

McMaster and co-workers[16] studied the effect of rubbing or spreading a cream on the skin using the guinea pig and rhesus monkey as animal models (Table 6). Cortisone was the test chemical and Feldmann and Maibach[1] had previously determined in man that the percutaneous absorption of cortisone (in acetone vehicle) was 3.4 ± 1.6% of applied dose. The absorption of cortisone spread on monkey skin was 5.3 ± 3.3% (similar to man) while that in the guinea pig was fourfold that of man and the rhesus monkey.

In general, the comparative in vivo data which have been reviewed demonstrate that percutaneous absorption in the pig and monkey (rhesus and squirrel) is in most cases similar to that in man, whereas in the rat, and especially in the rabbit, skin penetration is greater than that observed in man. The skin of the Mexican hairless dog has significantly different permeability characteristics than human skin. Absorption in the guinea pig was similar to man for hydrocortisone and benzoic acid, but high for testosterone and cortisone.

B. Comparative In Vitro Studies

Percutaneous absorption can be determined using the in vitro cell diffusion technique. Table 7 summarizes the ranking of skin permeability of different species, as determined in vitro by several investigators.[17-19] Allowing for the different compounds used in each study

Table 7
**RANKING OF SKIN
PERMEABILITY OF DIFFERENT
SPECIES AS DETERMINED IN
VITRO; LISTED IN DECREASING
ORDER OF PERMEABILITY**

Tregear[17]	Marzulli et al.[18]	McGreesh[19]
Rabbit	Mouse	Rabbit
Rat	Guinea pig	Rat
Guinea pig	Goat	Guinea pig
Man	Rabbit	Cat
	Horse	Goat
	Cat	Monkey
	Dog	Dog
	Monkey	Pig
	Weanling pig	
	Man	
	Chimpanzee	

to rank the species and the differences in origin of the skin sample (back forearm), the studies generally show that the skins of common laboratory animals (rabbit, rat, and guinea pig) are more permeable than the skin of man. Skins from the pig and the monkey more generally approximate the permeability of human skin. Not surprisingly, this general ranking is in close agreement with the in vivo data discussed earlier.

Campbell et al.[20] investigated the permeation of scopolamine in vitro through rat, rabbit, and human skin. The results indicated that human skin is the least permeable of the three species tested, and the relative order of rat and rabbit skin permeabilities depends both on skin location (back and side) and the method used to remove the hair.

In the study of Marzulli et al.[18] mouse skin was the most permeable, and was certainly much more permeable than human skin. In contrast, studies by Stoughton[21] using human and hairless mouse skin in vitro showed remarkable similarities in absorption for the skin of the two species for many compounds.

Table 8 summarizes the in vitro and in vivo percutaneous absorption of triclocarban (TCC) in adult (human and rhesus monkey) and newborn abdominal foreskin epidermis. The in vitro absorption using the static diffusion system was $0.23 \pm 0.15\%$ of applied dose for human adult abdominal skin. Similar results were obtained for newborn (0.26 ± 0.28), infant (0.29 ± 0.09), and adult rhesus abdominal skin (0.25 ± 0.09). The results suggest no difference in percutaneous absorption of these skin types.

Human newborn foreskin is used as a source of human skin for in vitro diffusion studies. The in vitro absorption for newborn foreskin was $2.5 \pm 1.6\%$. This was tenfold greater than human abdominal skin. Human adult foreskin absorption was $0.60 \pm 0.25\%$, suggesting that the newborn foreskin difference was possibly due to age (newborn) rather than site (foreskin), although probably both age and site contributed to the tenfold difference.

Another variable in an in vitro diffusion system is solubility of chemical in the receptor fluid. If the chemical diffusing through skin is not soluble in the receptor fluid, then diffusion is stopped and the chemical remains in the skin. This was ascertained for TCC which has high lipid solubility and low water solubility ($<50 \mu g/\ell$). In the static diffusion system set at room temperature (23°C), the absorption with human adult abdominal skin was $0.13 \pm 0.05\%$. With a continuous flow system absorption increased to $6.0 \pm 2.0\%$. The continuous flow system provides a larger sink (more volume) for the diffusing chemical to solubilize in. This is more analogous to the continual perfusion of blood and the in vivo situation. The percutaneous absorption of TCC in man was $7.0 \pm 2.8\%$. The continuous flow system

Table 8
IN VIVO AND IN VITRO PERCUTANEOUS
ABSORPTION OF TRICLOCARBAN IN ADULT
AND NEWBORN ABDOMINAL AND FORESKIN
EPIDERMIS

Skin type	Dose absorbed ± SD (%)
Static system 37°C	
Human adult abdominal (n = 14)	0.23 ± 0.15
Human newborn abdominal (n = 6)	0.26 ± 0.28
Human infant abdominal (n = 4)	0.29 ± 0.09
Monkey adult abdominal (n = 6)	0.25 ± 0.09
Human adult foreskin (n = 4)	0.60 ± 0.25
Human newborn foreskin (n = 7)	2.5 ± 1.6
Static system 23 ± C	
Human adult abdominal (n = 8)	0.13 ± 0.05
Continuous flow system 23 ± C	
Human adult abdominal (n = 12)	6.0 ± 2.0
Man *in vivo* (n = 5)	7.0 ± 2.8

From Wester, et al., *Percutaneous Absorption*, Bronough, R. and Maibach, H., Eds., Marcel Dekker, New York, 1985, 223. With permission.

and not the static diffusion system would be predictive of TCC in vivo percutaneous absorption in man.

Kligman[22] recently stated that in vitro data are more credible than in vivo data, and that if differences do exist then the in vivo data are suspect. Until recently the only comparative data available was the work of Franz[23] who evaluated the permeability of 12 organic compounds in vitro using excised human skin and compared the results to those obtained previously by Feldmann and Maibach in living man. Care was taken to ensure that his in vitro conditions closely followed those used in vivo, although it was necessary to use human abdominal skin for the in vitro studies. Additionally, the doses employed ranged from 4 to 40 μg/cm², with the assumption that the percent of applied dose absorbed would not be dose dependent. Quantitatively, the in vitro and in vivo data did not agree. The in vitro method was of value to the extent that it tended to distinguish compounds of low permeability from those of high permeability. However, there are notable differences such that the in vitro method alone would not always be a reliable or accurate predictor of percutaneous absorption in living man. Franz[24] further evaluated the finite dose methodology and got closer correlation between in vitro and in vivo data.

Table 9 gives the in vivo and in vitro dermal absorption of paraquat and water through human and laboratory animal skin. The permeability rate of paraquat through human skin was some tenfold less in vivo than in vitro. Comparison of in vitro permeability constants for water and paraquat show that most laboratory animal skin is not predictive of human skin.

Table 9 on paraquat absorption and Table 8 on triclocarban absorption give additional in vivo/in vitro comparison for human skin. For each chemical the difference was at least tenfold. With triclocarban the difference was due to the in vitro diffusion cell mechanism where the chemical was not soluble in the low volume of diffusion media. This was corrected with a continuous flow system and of in vivo absorption. Until these in vivo/in vitro discrepancies cease to appear, in vivo determinations must be continued and the in vitro systems remain as experimental models, urgently needing further validation for relevance to man.

Table 9
IN VIVO AND IN VITRO ABSORPTION OF PARAQUAT AND WATER THROUGH HUMAN AND LABORATORY ANIMAL SKIN

In vivo/in vitro specie	Paraquat Permeability rate ($\mu g/cm^2$)
Human (in vivo)[31]	0.03
Human (in vitro)[32]	0.5

In vitro [33] specie	Permeability constant (cm/hr $\times$ 10^5)	
	Water	Paraquat
Human	93	0.7
Rat	103	27.2
Hairless rat	130	35.3
Nude rat	152	35.5[a]
Mouse	164	97.2[a]
Hairless mouse	254[a]	1065.0[a]
Rabbit	253[a]	92.9[a]
Guinea pig	442[a]	196.0[a]

[a]   Significantly different from human.

Table 10
HUMAN AND ANIMAL SKIN THICKNESS MEASUREMENTS

Type of skin	Stratum corneum (μm)	Epidermis (μm)	Whole skin (mm)
Human (16)	16.8 ± 0.7	46.9 ± 2.3	2.97 ± 0.28
Pig (35)	26.4 ± 0.4	65.8 ± 1.8	3.43 ± 0.05
Rat (9)	18.4 ± 0.5	32.1 ± 1.3	2.09 ± 0.07
Hairless Mouse (12)	8.9 ± 0.4	28.6 ± 0.9	0.70 ± 0.02
Mouse (9)	5.8 ± 0.3	12.6 ± 0.8	0.84 ± 0.02

Note: Values are means $\pm$ SE of the thickness of the number of sections in parentheses. Three to six sections were taken from each skin sample.

From Bronaugh, R. L., et al., *Toxicol. Appl. Pharmacol.*, 62, 481, 1982. With permission.

II. DISCUSSION

The overriding theory of percutaneous absorption has been Fick's law of diffusion and it has been used to explain all aspects of percutaneous absorption including specie differences. Fick's law would account for specie differences by the differences in skin thickness.[22] However, measurements of skin thickness such as in Table 10 do not correlate with specie differences in percutaneous absorption.[25] A theory presented by Elias and co-workers[26,27] is that the lipid content of skin represents the barrier to percutaneous absorption and that differences in species (or other aspects such as site variation) are due to differences in lipid content.

In reviewing studies comparing percutaneous absorption between animals and man, care must be taken to ascertain what influences the methodology may have had on the data. Differences in results can be due to different techniques used in the study. This becomes very important when the data from animal study are compared to published literature values on absorption in man. Subtle differences in technology may not be readily expressed in the printed methodology.

When comparing the percutaneous absorption of species it becomes obvious that differences do exist. Some of these differences are due to the species themselves and some of the differences are due to techniques used in the study. Various parameters can also affect percutaneous absorption.[28,29] It becomes important that in any species comparative study, the methods and techniques used must be as close to each other as possible. Some of the parameters such as site of application, occlusion, dose concentration, surface area, and vehicle can be controlled by the investigator. Some parameters such as skin metabolism, skin age, and skin condition may, in part, be difficult for an investigator to control.

The perfect comparative study probably cannot be done, however, the data in the literature suggest that differences in percutaneous absorption exist between species. Compared to absorption in man, absorption in common laboratory animals, rats, and rabbits, is high. Absorption in the pig and the monkey (squirrel and rhesus) appears more predictive of that in vivo, the comparative in vitro studies done with skin from different species favorably agree with the in vivo results.

Thus, it appears that the animal models most predictive of percutaneous absorption for predicting transdermal delivery in man are the pig and monkey. However, this does not mean that the investigator does meaningless studies in vitro or in vivo with rats and rabbits; what it means is that the results obtained must be carefully explained within the scope of the methods and species used. Correlations and predictions of results to man must be done with utmost care.

REFERENCES

1. **Feldmann, R. J. and Maibach, H. I.,** Percutaneous penetration of steroids in man, *J. Invest. Dermatol.,* 52, 89, 1969.
2. **Feldmann, R. J. and Maibach, H. I.,** Absorption of some organic compounds through the skin in man, *J. Invest. Dermatol.,* 54, 339, 1969.
3. **Feldmann, R. J. and Maibach, H. I.,** Percutaneous penetration of some pesticides and herbicides in man, *Toxicol. Appl. Pharmacol.,* 28, 126, 1974.
4. **Bartek, M. J., LaBudde, J. A., and Maibach, H. I.,** Skin permeability in vivo: comparison in rat, rabbit, pig, and man, *J. Invest. Dermatol.,* 58, 114, 1972.
5. **Bartek, M. J. and La Budde, J. A.,** Percutaneous absorption in vitro, in *Animal Models in Dermatology: Relevance to Human Dermatopharmacology and Dermatotoxicology,* Maibach, H., Ed., Churchill Livingstone, London, 1975, 103.
6. **Wester, R. C. and Maibach, H. I.,** Percutaneous absorption in the rhesus monkey compared to man, *Toxicol. Appl. Pharmacol.,* 32, 394, 1975.
7. **Wester, R. C. and Maibach, H. I.,** Rhesus monkey as an animal model for percutaneous absorption, in *Animal Models in Dermatology: Relevance to Human Dermatopharmacology and Dermatotoxicology,* Maibach, H., Ed., Churchill Livingstone, London, 1975, 133.
8. **Wester, R. C. and Maibach, H. I.,** Relationship of topical dose and percutaneous absorption in rhesus monkey and man, *J. Invest. Dermatol.,* 67, 518, 1976.
9. **Wester, R. C. and Maibach, H. I.,** Percutaneous absorption in man and animal: a perspective, *Cutaneous Toxicity,* Drill, V. and Lazar, P., Eds., Academic Press, New York, 1977, 111.
10. **Wester, R. C., Noonan, P. K., and Maibach, H. I.,** Recent advances in percutaneous absorption using the rhesus monkey model, *J. Soc. Cosmet. Chem.,* 30, 297, 1979.
11. **Andersen, K. E., Maibach, H. I., and Ango, M. D.,** The guinea pig: an animal model for human skin absorption of hydrocortisone, testosterone and, benzoic acid?, *Br. J. Dermatol.,* 102, 447, 1980.

12. **Wester, R. C. and Noonan, P. K.,** Topical bioavailability of a potential anti-acne agent (SC-23110) as determined by cumulative excretion and areas under plasma concentration-time curves, *J. Invest. Dermatol.*, 70, 92, 1978.

13. **Hunziker, N., Feldmann, R. J., and Maibach, H. I.,** Animal models of percutaneous penetration: comparison in Mexican hairless dogs and man, *Dermatologica*, 156, 79, 1978.

14. **Feldmann, R. J. and Maibach, H. I.,** Regional variation in percutaneous penetration of ^{14}C-cortisone in man, *J. Invest. Dermatol.*, 48, 181, 1967.

15. **Wester, R. C., Noonan, P. K., and Maibach, H. I.,** Variations in percutaneous absorption of testosterone in the rhesus monkey due to anatomic site of application and frequency of application, *Arch. Dermatol. Res.*, 267, 229, 1980.

16. **McMaster, J., Maibach, H. I., Wester, R. C., and Bucks, D.,** Does rubbing enhance in vivo dermal absorption?, personal communication.

17. **Tregear, R. T.,** *Physical Function of Skin*, Academic Press, New York, 1966.

18. **Marzulli, F. N., Brown, D. W. C., and Maibach, H. I.,** Techniques for studying skin penetration, *Toxicol. Appl. Pharmacol., Suppl*, 3, 79, 1969.

19. **McGreesh, A. H.,** Percutaneous toxicity, *Toxicol. Appl. Pharmacol., Suppl.*, 2, 20, 1965.

20. **Campbell, P., Watanabe, T., and Chandrasekaran, S. K.,** Comparison of *in vitro* skin permeability of scopolamine in rat, rabbit, and man, *Fed. Proc. Fed. Am. Soc. Exp. Biol.*, 35, 639, 1976.

21. **Stoughton, R. B.,** Animal models for *in vitro* percutaneous absorption, in *Animal Models in Dermatology: Relevance to Human Dermatopharmacology and Dermatotoxicology*, Maibach, H., Ed., Churchill Livingstone, London, 1975, 121.

22. **Kligman, A. M.,** A biological brief on percutaneous absorption, *Drug Dev. Indust. Pharm.*, 521, 1983.

23. **Franz, T. J.,** Percutaneous absorption. On the relevance of *in vitro* data, *J. Invest. Dermatol.*, 64, 190, 1975.

24. **Franz, T. J.,** The finite dose technique as a valid *in vitro* model for study of percutaneous absorption in man, Annual Scientific Seminar, Soc. Cosmet. Chem., Dallas, May, 1979.

25. **Bronaugh, R. L., Stewart, R. F., and Cougdon, E. R.,** Methods for *in vitro* percutaneous absorption studies. II. Animal models for human skin, *Toxicol. Appl. Pharmacol.*, 62, 481, 1982.

26. **Elias, P. M., Brown, B. E., and Ziboh, V. A.,** The permeability barrier in essential fatty acid deficiency: evidence for a direct role for linoleic acid in barrier function, *J. Invest. Dermatol.*, 73, 230, 1980.

27. **Elias, P. M., Cooper, E. R., Korc, A., and Brown, B. E.,** Percutaneous transport in relation to stratum corneum structure and lipid composition, *J. Invest. Dermatol.*, 76, 297, 1981.

28. **Wester, R. C. and Maibach, H. I.,** Cutaneous pharmacokinetics: 10 steps to percutaneous absorption, *Drug Metab. Rev.*, 14, 169, 1983.

29. **Wester, R. C. and Noonan, P. K.,** Relevance of animal models for percutaneous absorption, *Int. J. Pharm.*, 7, 99, 1980.

30. **Wester, R. C., Maibach, H. I., Surinchak, J., and Bucks, D. A. W.,** Predictability of *in vitro* diffusion systems and skin types and ages on percutaneous absorption of triclocarban, in *Percutaneous Absorption*, Bronough, R. and Maibach, H., Eds, Marcel Dekker, New York, 1985, 223.

31. **Wester, R. C., Maibach, H. I., Bucko, D. A. W., and Aufrere, M. B.,** *In vivo* percutaneous absorption of paraquat from hands, legs, and forearm of man, *J. Toxicol. Environ. Health*, (in press, 1984).

32. **Dugard, P. H.,** personal communication, 1984.

33. **Walker, M., Dugard, P. H., and Scott, R. C.,** *In vitro* percutaneous absorption studies: a comparison of human and laboratory species, *Human Toxicol.*, 2, 561, 1983.

Chapter 6

CLINICAL CONSIDERATIONS FOR TRANSDERMAL DELIVERY

Ronald C. Wester and Howard I. Maibach

TABLE OF CONTENTS

I. INTRODUCTION

There are two major parts to transdermal drug delivery, the transdermal device and the skin. The device is the hardware which will be manipulated and outfitted with various controlled release potentials for a variety of drugs. In contrast, the skin is an evolutionary masterpiece of living tissue which is the final control unit for determining the systemic availability of any drug which must pass through it. Thus, those parameters which skin has for controlling percutaneous absorption are important because all transdermal drugs and devices must be subjected to them. The following is a discussion of some parameters of clinical percutaneous absorption which are important to transdermal drug delivery.

A. In Vivo Methodology

Percutaneous absorption in vivo is usually determined by the indirect method of measuring radioactivity in excreta following topical application of the labeled compound. In human studies, plasma levels of compounds are extremely low following topical application, often below assay detection level, so it is necessary to use tracer methodology. The labeled compound, usually carbon-14 or tritium, is applied and the total amount of radioactivity excreted in urine or urine plus feces determined. The amount of radioactivity retained in the body or excreted by some route not assayed (CO_2 and sweat) is corrected for by determining the amount of radioactivity excreted following parenteral administration. This final amount of radioactivity is then expressed as the percent of applied dose which was absorbed.

The equation used to determine percutaneous absorption is

$$\text{Percent} = \frac{\text{Total radioactivity following topical administration}}{\text{Total radioactivity following parenteral administration}} \times 100$$

Determination of percutaneous absorption from urinary radioactivity excretion does not account for metabolism by skin. The radioactivity in urine is usually a mixture of the parent compound and metabolites. Plasma radioactivity can be measured and the percutaneous absorption determined by the ratio of the areas under the plasma vs. time concentration curves following topical and intravenous administration. Note that radioactivity in blood and excreta can include both the applied compound and metabolites. If the metabolism by the skin is extensive and different from that of other systemic tissues, then this method is not valid because the pharmacokinetics of the metabolites can be different from that of the parent compound. However, in actual practice, the plasma assay method has given results similar to those obtained from urinary excretion.

The only way to determine the absolute bioavailability of a topically applied compound is to measure the compound by specific assay in blood or urine following topical and intravenous administration. This may be extremely difficult to do because plasma concentrations after topical administration are often low. However, as analytical methodology brings forth more sensitive assays, estimates of absolute topical bioavailability will become a reality.

A comparative example of the above three methods was done using [^{14}C]nitroglycerin in the rhesus monkey (Table 1). Topical bioavailability estimated from urinary excretion was 72.7 ± 5.8%. This was similar to the 77.2 ± 6.7% estimated from plasma total radioactivity AUC (area under plasma concentration vs. time curve). The absolute bioavailability estimated from plasma nitroglycerin unchanged compound AUCs was 56.6 ± 2.5%. The estimates from plasma ^{14}C and urinary ^{14}C were in good agreement. Also, the difference in estimate between that of the absolute bioavailability (56%) and that of ^{14}C (72.7 to 77.2%) may be the percent of compound metabolized in the skin as the compound was being absorbed. For nitroglycerin this is about 20%.[1]

Another approach taken to determine in vivo percutaneous absorption is to determine the

Table 1
BIOAVAILABILITY OF TOPICAL
NITROGLYCERIN DETERMINED FROM
PLASMA NITROGLYCERIN, PLASMA ^{14}C,
AND URINARY EXCRETION OF ^{14}C[a]

Method	Mean bioavailability (%)
Plasma nitroglycerin AUC[a]	56.6 ± 2.5
Plasma total radioactivity AUC[a]	77.2 ± 6.7
Urinary total radioactivity[b]	72.7 ± 5.8

[a] Absolute bioavailability of nitroglycerin:

$$\text{Percent} = \frac{[\text{AUC (ng} \cdot \text{h} \cdot \text{m}\ell^{-1})]/[\text{topical dose}]}{[\text{AUC (ng} \cdot \text{h} \cdot \text{m}\ell^{-1})]/[\text{i.v. dose}]} \times 100$$

[b] Absolute bioavailability of ^{14}C:

$$^{b}\text{Percent} = \frac{\text{Total } ^{14}\text{C excretion following topical administration}}{\text{Total } ^{14}\text{C excretion following i.v. administration}} \times 100$$

From Wester, R. C., et al., *J. Pharm. Sci.*, 72, 745, 1983. With permission.

loss of material from the surface as it penetrates into the skin. Skin recovery from an ointment or solution application is difficult because total recovery of compound from the skin is never assured. With topical application of a transdermal delivery device, the total unit can be removed from the skin and the residual amount of drug in the device determined. It is assumed that the difference between applied dose and residual dose is the amount of drug absorbed.

Another in vivo method of estimating absorption is to use a biological/pharmacological response. There, biological assay is substituted for a chemical assay and absorption is estimated. An obvious disadvantage of the use of biological responses is that they are limited to compounds which elicit responses that can be measured easily and accurately. An example of a biological response would be the vasoconstrictor assay when the blanching effect of one compound is compared to a known compound. This method is more qualitative than quantitative, and may confuse the effects of differences in transport with differences in biological interactions.

Other qualitative methods of estimating in vivo percutaneous absorption include whole-body autoradiography and fluorescence. Whole-body autoradiography provides an overall picture of the dermal absorption followed by the involvement of other body tissues.

B. Individual Variation

The percutaneous absorption of hydrocortisone was studied in 18 healthy adult males.[2] The anatomic site was the same, as was the dose (4 μg/cm^2). The mean absorption was 0.9% of the applied dose. However, the absorption for several individuals was one third as much, whereas one subject absorbed three times more than the median. Thus, there was a tenfold difference in the range. The variation was as might be expected in almost any biological system. Thus, there can be a severalfold difference in absorption even when the site of application, dose, vehicle, etc., is the same.

Table 2
PERCUTANEOUS
ABSORPTION OF
HYDROCORTISONE
THROUGH MODIFIED SKIN

Treatment	Penetration ratio
None	1
Strip	4
Occlude	10
Cantharidine blister	15
Strip + occlude	20

From Feldmann, R. J. and Maibach, H.
I., *J. Invest. Dermatol.*, 48, 181, 1967.
With permission.

C. Skin Condition

There are skin conditions other than hydration and temperature which affect percutaneous absorption. The most obvious condition is loss of barrier function of the stratum corneum through disease or damage. Skin condition also changes with age. The genesis of the stratum corneum occurs during gestation and is probably concluded at birth. Preterm infants probably do not have a fully developed stratum corneum and therefore have increased skin permeability. Skin of the elderly also undergoes changes which can influence absorption. Virtually any type of change in skin condition, especially change in the barrier function of the stratum corneum, whether natural or inflicted, will affect percutaneous absorption.

Damage, disease, and local conditions may increase the absorption of compounds to levels much greater than those observed for normal skin. Shown in Table 2 are the results of the following modifications: removal of the stratum corneum with cellophane tape stripping, occlusion with plastic film, removal of the epidermis with a cantharidine solution, and the combination of stripping and occlusion.[3] Stripping the skin with tape until it glistens removes the stratum corneum and causes damage to the upper layers of the epidermis; this procedure is often used as a model for damaged and diseased skin. Stripped skin shows a fourfold increase in penetration of hydrocortisone. Occluding the hydrocortisone with a plastic film during the first 24 hr causes a tenfold increase in absorption over unoccluded skin. Recent unpublished work at our laboratory indicates that trapping of water under the occlusive layer is necessary for this increased penetration. Removal of the epidermis with topical application of a cantharidine solution leaves a denuded skin site which absorbs 15 times more hydrocortisone than untreated skin. The greatest absorption was obtained by stripping following by a 24-hr occlusion, yielding penetration 20 times the value for normal skin.

It is commonly stated that the stratum corneum is the barrier to percutaneous penetration; this appears generally true for intact skin. Fortunately, when the stratum corneum is damaged, the other layers function as barriers to penetration; as evidenced by these data, none of the damages inflicted upon the skin caused 100% penetration. Presumably each epidermal cell membrane, the basement membrane, and other cellular structures have substantial barrier properties to hydrocortisone.

D. Skin Site of Application

The extent of absorption depends upon the anatomical site to which the compound is applied. This is true for both man[4,5] and animals.[6,7] Presented in Table 3 are data derived from in vivo absorptions of hydrocortisone after application to various human anatomic

Table 3
REGIONAL VARIATION IN
PERCUTANEOUS
ABSORPTION OF
HYDROCORTISONE IN MAN

Site of application	Absorption ratio
Forearm (ventral)	1.1 ×
Forearm (dorsal)	1.1 ×
Foot arch (plantar)	0.14 ×
Ankle (lateral)	0.42 ×
Palm	0.83 ×
Back	1.7 ×
Scalp	3.5 ×
Axilla	3.6 ×
Forehead	6.0 ×
Jaw angle	13.0 ×
Scrotum	42.0 ×

From Maibach, H. I., et al., *Arch. Environ. Health*, 23, 208, 1971. With permission.

sites.[5] They are of obvious practical significance in that high total absorption is found for head, neck, and axilla, where both cosmetic and environmental exposure are greater. Preliminary results show that the female genitalia show greater absorption than forearm skin surfaces (not mucosa), but not so great as scrotal skin. Similar results in anatomical variation have been shown for pesticides.[4] With a wide variety of chemical moieties examined (steroids, pesticides, and antimicrobials), the general pattern of regional variation holds. One important exception is carbaryl, which was extensively absorbed from the forearm, although the other sites were not significantly higher. This finding suggests that carbaryl is extensively absorbed from all body sites.

For transdermal delivery this has presented a problem because patient compliance would probably be better if the patient had a choice of where to apply the transdermal unit. Changing skin sites daily also avoids the question of constant occlusion/adhesive in the same site altering absorption. Further study and clinical experience will determine whether this is a problem in transdermal delivery.

E. Occlusion

Transdermal units by nature of their design occlude the site of application. This is important for drug delivery because percutaneous absorption is increased when the site of application is occluded. Occlusion is a covering of the applied dose, either intentionally, as with bandaging, or unintentionally, as putting on clothing after applying a topical compound. A vehicle such as an ointment can also have occlusive properties. Occlusion results in a combination of many physical factors affecting skin and the applied compound. Occlusion changes the hydration and temperature of the skin, and these physical factors affect absorption. Occlusion also prevents the accidental wiping or evaporation (volatile compound) of the applied compound, in essence maintaining a higher applied dose. For hydrocortisone, there is more percutaneous absorption with occlusion than even with stripping (Table 2). Occlusion is also the most practical clinical method to enhance percutaneous absorption. It should be remembered that any attempt to design transdermal units without occlusive properties (air vents, etc.) would remove the enhancing absorption properties that occlusion has.

Behl et al.[8] showed that hydration of the skin increased penetration of lipid-soluble, nonpolar molecules but had less effect on the penetration of polar molecules. Many drugs

Table 4
APPARENT TRANSDERMAL ABSORPTION RATES OF NITROGLYCERIN IN HEALTHY VOLUNTEERS

	Absorption rate (μg/hr/cm^2)		
Volunteer	Nitro-Bid®	Nitro-Dur®	Nitrodisc®
D.D.	4.72	2.34	3.45
M.D.	6.95	9.90	3.37
T.M.(1)	4.12	3.78	5.51
T.M.(2)	4.87	—	—
J.K.	—	16.3	—
R.D.	5.08	—	9.86
Mean	5.15	8.09	5.55
± SD	1.07	6.35	3.04
% CV	20.8	78.4	54.8

From Noonan, et al., *10th Int. Symp. Controlled Rel. Bioact. Mater.*, 1983, 332. With permission.

belong to this first category, and scientists have recognized that hydration increases penetration because occlusion increases penetration and causes endogenous hydration of the stratum corneum.

The reservoir effect is an example of change in penetration rates as a result of hydration. Initially, a drug applied under occlusion enters the stratum corneum. When the occlusive dressing is removed and the stratum corneum dehydrates, the movement of drug slows and the stratum corneum becomes a reservoir. Subsequently, occlusion alone will hydrate the tissue and increase the rate of movement of drug, and its pharmacological action again becomes apparent.

F. Defining Clinical Dose

Table 4 gives the apparent transdermal absorption rates of nitroglycerin in healthy volunteers administered nitroglycerin in an ointment (Nitro-Bid®) and transdermal devices (Nitro-Dur® and Nitrodisc®).[9] Absorption rates for the same drug in various dosage forms are important for the clinician to know so that one dosage form may be (or may not be) substituted for another.

There are two parts to bioavailability, the rate as shown above, and the total dose absorbed (usually expressed as percent of applied dose). It is also important for the clinician to know the total dose which is delivered systemically. With transdermal delivery/percutaneous absorption there are some important factors in the dosage form which define the dose. These are (1) total dose, (2) surface area, (3) concentration, and (4) time of application.

1. **Total dose** — This is the total amount of drug in the transdermal unit which is potentially available for systemic delivery.
2. **Surface area** — Systemic availability of a transdermal drug can be increased with a changing surface area. However, consumer acceptance will limit the size of the transdermal devices. Table 5 shows the interaction of surface area and concentrations on the ability of the skin to efficiently absorb nitroglycerin. For a constant dose (40 mg), the surface area will determine concentration per unit of the skin area, and this will determine the efficiency of skin absorption.[10]

Table 5
SURFACE AREA AND NITROGLYCERIN
PERCUTANEOUS ABSORPTION

Total dose (mg)	Surface area	Concentration (mg/cm^2)	Dose absorbed (%)
40	2 cm	20	13.4 ± 1.2
40	50 cm^2	0.8	36.4 ± 4.3

From Wester, R. C., *10th Symp. Controlled Rel. Bioact. Mater.*, 1983, 329. With permission.

Table 6
EFFECT OF CONCENTRATION
ON PERCUTANEOUS
ABSORPTION OF
NITROGLYCERIN

Nitroglycerin concentration (mg/cm^2)	Dose absorbed (%)	Total mg absorbed
0.01	41.8	0.004
0.1	43.5	0.04
1.0	36.6	0.4
7.0	26.8	1.9
10.0	7.8	0.8

From Wester, R. C., *10th Int. Symp. Controlled Rel. Bioact. Mater.*, 1983, 329. With permission.

3. **Concentration (total dose/surface area = concentration)** — Table 6 gives the percutaneous absorption in the rhesus monkey for increasing concentrations of nitroglycerin applied as ethanolic solutions to a constant surface area for 24 hr. The percent dose absorbed was fairly constant over the range of 0.01 to 1.0 mg/cm^2. However, for 7 and 10 mg/cm^2, the efficiency of absorption decreased, suggesting a saturation of the skin's absorption processes. Thus, the total dose on a given area can limit absorption.[10]

4. **Time** — Table 7 gives the effect of time (duration of being on skin) on percutaneous absorption of malathion (under occlusion) in man.[11] The longer the chemical was on the skin, the greater the absorption (systemic availability) became.

Thus, a transdermal unit defines total dose, surface area, and concentration of drug. These factors plus time of skin application have a large effect on the bioavailability (rate and percent dose absorbed) of a drug in man.

II. DISCUSSION

Our message here is a simple one. Of the two parts to transdermal delivery, device and skin, the skin will have the final say in determining bioavailability and clinical acceptance. The absorption of the skin will be influenced by formulations and designs in the device. The skin will then respond because it is a living tissue, and this response will determine the toxicity and efficacy of the transdermal system.

Table 7
EFFECT OF TIME ON
PERCUTANEOUS
ABSORPTION OF
MALATHION

Time (hr)	Dose absorbed (%)
0	9.6
0.5	7.3
1	12.7
2	16.6
4	24.2
8	38.8
24	62.8

From Maibach, H. I. and Feldmann, R.,
Occupational Exposure to Pesticides:
Report to the Federal Working Group on
Pest Management, 1974, 120. With
permission.

REFERENCES

1. **Wester, R. C., Noonan, P. K., Smeach, S., and Kosobud, L.,** Pharmacokinetics and bioavailability of intravenous and topical nitroglycerin in the rhesus monkey. Estimate of percutaneous first-pass metabolism, *J. Pharm. Sci.,* 72, 745, 1983.
2. **Maibach, H. I.,** In vivo percutaneous penetration of corticoids in man and unresolved problems in their efficacy, *Dermatologica, Suppl.,* 152, 11, 1976.
3. **Feldmann, R. J. and Maibach, H. I.,** Penetration of ^{14}C hydrocortisone through normal skin, *Arch. Dermatol.,* 91, 661, 1965.
4. **Maibach, H. I., Feldmann, R. J., Milby, T. H., and Serat, W. F.,** Regional variation in percutaneous penetration in man, *Arch. Environ. Health,* 23, 208, 1971.
5. **Feldmann, R. J. and Maibach, H. I.,** Regional variation in percutaneous penetration of ^{14}C cortisol in man, *J. Invest. Dermatol.,* 48, 181, 1967.
6. **Wester, R. C., Noonan, P. K., and Maibach, H. I.,** Variations in percutaneous absorption of testosterone in the rhesus monkey due to anatomic site of application and frequency of application, *Arch. Dermatol. Res.,* 267, 229, 1980.
7. **Noonan, P. K. and Wester, R. C.,** Percutaneous absorption of nitroglycerin, *J. Pharm. Sci.,* 69, 385, 1980.
8. **Behl, C. R., Flynn, G. L., Kurihara, T., Harper, N., Smith, W., Higuchi, W. I., Ho, N. F. H., and Pierson, C. L.,** Hydration and percutaneous absorption. I. Influence of hydration on alkanol permeation through hairless mouse skin, *J. Invest. Dermatol.,* 75, 346, 1980.
9. **Noonan, P. K., Rigod, J. F., Williams, R. L., and Benet, L. Z.,** Transdermal absorption rates of nitroglycerin in healthy volunteers, 10th Int. Symp. Controlled Rel. Bioact. Mater., 1983, 332.
10. **Wester, R. C.,** Role of skin in nitroglycerin transdermal delivery, 10th Int. Symp. Controlled Rel. Bioact. Mater., 1983, 329.
11. **Maibach, H. I. and Feldmann, R.,** Systemic absorption of pesticides through the skin of man, in *Occupational Exposure to Pesticides: Report to the Federal Working Group on Pest Management*, Appendix B., 1974, 120.

Section III: Devices

Chapter 7

DEVELOPMENT OF TRANSDERMAL CONTROLLED RELEASE DRUG DELIVERY SYSTEMS: AN OVERVIEW

Yie W. Chien

TABLE OF CONTENTS

I. INTRODUCTION

For many decades, the skin has been commonly used as the site for the administration of dermatological drugs to achieve a localized pharmacologic action in the skin. In this case, the drug molecule is considered to diffuse to a target tissue in the vicinity of drug application to produce its therapeutic effect before it is distributed to the systemic circulation for elimination (Figure 1). It is exemplified by the use of hydrocortisone for dermatitis, benzoyl peroxide for acne, and neomycin for superficial infection.[4]

Most recently, there is an increasing recognition that the skin can also serve as the port of administration for systemically active drugs (Figure 1). In this case, the drug which is applied topically will be absorbed first into the blood circulation and then be transported to target tissues, which is distant from the site of drug administration, to achieve its therapeutic purposes. It is exemplified by the transdermal administration of nitroglycerin for the treatment of angina pectoris, of scopolamine for the prevention of motion sickness, and of estradiol for the medication of postmenopause.[5-7] This chapter intends to provide an overview on the development of drug delivery systems (transdermal therapeutic systems or patches) for the transdermal controlled administration of drugs for systemic medications.

II. FUNDAMENTALS OF SKIN PERMEATION

For a systemically active drug to reach a target tissue remote from the site of drug administration on the skin surface, it has to possess some physicochemical properties which facilitate the sorption of drug by the stratum corneum, the penetration of drug through various skin tissues, and also the uptake of the drug by the capillary network in the dermal papillary layer (Figure 2). The steady-state rate of permeation, dQ/dt, across the skin can be expressed, mathematically, by the following relationship:[8]

$$\frac{dQ}{dt} = P_s (C_d - C_r) \tag{1}$$

Where C_d and C_r are, respectively, the concentrations of a skin penetrant in the donor compartment, e.g., the drug concentration on the surface of stratum corneum, and in the receptor compartment, e.g., body; and P_s is the permeability coefficient of the skin as defined by:

$$P_s = \frac{K_s D_{ss}}{h_s} \tag{2}$$

Where K_s is the partition coefficient for the interfacial partitioning of the penetrant molecule from a transdermal drug delivery system onto the skin tissues; D_{ss} is the diffusivity for the steady-state diffusion of the penetrant molecule through the skin tissues; and h_s is the total thickness of the skin tissues. The skin permeability coefficient (P_s) for a skin penetrant can be considered as a constant since K_s, D_{ss}, and h_s terms in Equation 2 are constant values under a fixed condition.

Analysis of Equation 1 suggests that in order to achieve a constant rate of drug permeation, it requires a condition being maintained that the drug concentration on the surface of stratum corneum (C_d) is consistently and substantially greater than the drug concentration in the body (C_r), i.e., $C_d >> C_r$; therefore, Equation 1 can be reduced to:

$$\frac{dQ}{dt} = P_s C_d \tag{3}$$

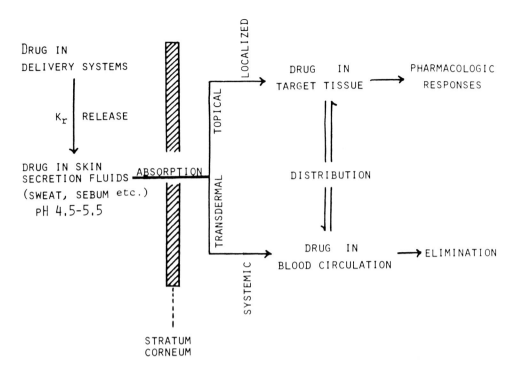

FIGURE 1. Percutaneous absorption of drugs for localized therapeutic actions in the skin tissues or for systemic medications in the tissues remote from the site of topical drug application.

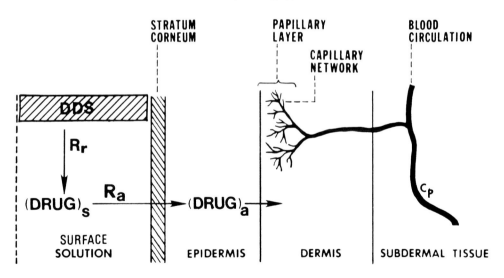

FIGURE 2. Diagrammatic illustration of the relationship between the rate of drug release (R_r) from a transdermal drug delivery system and the rate of drug uptake (R_a) by the skin.

and the rate of skin permeation (dQ/dt) becomes a constant, since the C_d value remains fairly constant throughout the course of skin permeation. To maintain the C_d at a constant value, it is critical to release the drug at a rate (R_r) which is always greater than the rate of skin transport (R_a), i.e., $R_r \gg R_a$ (Figure 2). By doing that, the drug concentration on the skin surface is maintained at a level which is always greater than the equilibrium (or

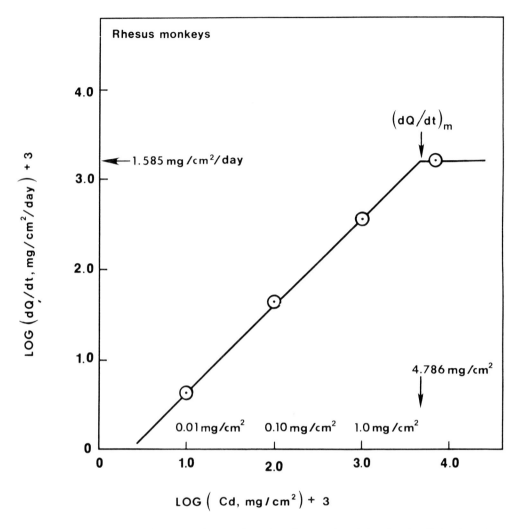

FIGURE 3. Linear relationship between the rate of transdermal permeation of nitroglycerin (dQ/dt), determined from the daily urinary recovery data, and the nitroglycerin dose applied on the rhesus monkey skin (C_d)[9].

saturation) solubility in the stratum corneum, i.e., $C_d \gg C_s^e$, and a maximum rate of skin permeation, $(dQ/dt)_m$, is reached as expressed by:

$$\left(\frac{dQ}{dt}\right)_m = P_s C_s^e \qquad (4)$$

The magnitude of $(dQ/dt)_m$ is thus determined by the skin permeability coefficient (P_s) of the drug and its equilibrium solubility in the stratum corneum (C_s^e). This concept of stratum corneum-limited skin permeation was investigated by depositing various doses of pure, radiolabeled nitroglycerin, in a volatile organic solvent, onto a controlled skin surface area of rhesus monkeys.[9] Results from the urinary recovery data indicated that the rate of skin permeation (dQ/dt) increases as increasing the nitroglycerin dose (C_d) applied on a unity surface area of the skin (Figure 3). It appears that a maximum rate of skin permeation (1.585 mg/cm²/day) is reached for nitroglycerin when the applied dose achieves the level of 4.786 mg/cm². It translates into a maximum transdermal bioavailability of 33.1% per day.

The kinetics of skin permeation can be more precisely analyzed by studying the time

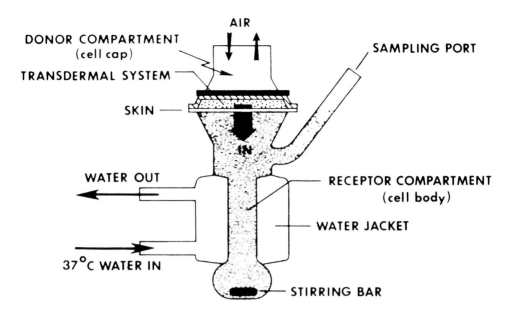

FIGURE 4. Diagrammatic illustration of one unit of the commercially available 8-cell Franz diffusion apparatus (Reproduced from Crown Glass Co., Inc., Somerville, N. J.).

course for the permeation of drug across a freshly excised skin mounted on a diffusion cell, such as the Franz diffusion cell (Figure 4). A typical skin permeation kinetic profile is shown in Figure 5 for nitroglycerin. Results indicated that at an applied dose of 14.32 mg/cm^2, nitroglycerin penetrates through the hairless mouse skin at a zero-order rate of 19.85 ($\pm$ 1.71) μg/cm^2/hr. Pure nitroglycerin (without the organic solvent) was used in this investigation.[10]

III. APPROACHES FOR CONTROLLED SKIN PERMEATION

Several technologies have been developed to provide a rate-control over the release and the skin permeation of drugs. These technologies can be classified into four approaches as outlined in the following.

A. Membrane-Moderated Transdermal Drug Delivery Systems

In this approach, the drug reservoir is totally encapsulated in a shallow compartment molded from a drug-impermeable metallic plastic laminate and a rate-controlling polymeric membrane (Figure 6). The drug molecules are permitted to release only through the rate-controlling membrane. In the drug reservoir compartment, the drug solids are dispersed in a solid polymer matrix or suspended in an unleachable, viscous liquid medium to form a paste-like suspension. The rate-limiting membrane can be a microporous or a nonporous polymeric membrane with a defined drug permeability property. On the external surface of the polymeric membrane, a thin layer of drug-compatible, hypoallergenic adhesive polymer may be applied to achieve an intimate contact of the transdermal patch with the skin. The rate of drug release from this type of transdermal drug delivery system can be tailored by varying the polymer composition, permeability coefficient, and thickness of the rate-limiting membrane and adhesive. Several transdermal therapeutic systems have been successfully developed from this technology and are best exemplified by the development of Transderm-Nitro® system (Ciba Pharmaceutical Co., Summit, N.J.) for once-a-day medication of angina pectoris,[11,12] and of Transderm Scōp® system for 3-day protection of motion sickness.[13] The system components of Transderm-Nitro® system and some of their physical properties are outlined in Table 1.

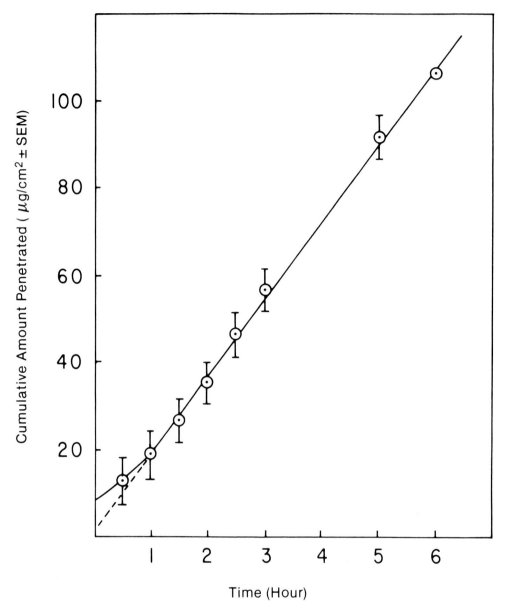

FIGURE 5.   Permeation profile of pure nitroglycerin across hairless mouse abdominal skin mounted on Franz diffusion apparatus at 37°C. A constant skin permeation profile was obtained with a permeation rate of 19.85 (±1.71) μg/cm²/hr.[10]

The intrinsic rate of drug release from this type of drug delivery system is defined by:

$$\frac{dQ}{dt} = \frac{C_R}{\frac{1}{P_m} + \frac{1}{P_a}} \tag{5}$$

Where C_R is the drug concentration in the reservoir compartment, P_a and P_m are the permeability coefficients of the adhesive layer and the rate-controlling membrane, respectively. For a microporous membrane, P_m is approximately the sum of permeability coefficients across the pores and the polymeric material.[14] P_m and P_a, respectively, are defined as follows:

MEMBRANE-MODERATED
TRANSDERMAL DRUG DELIVERY SYSTEMS

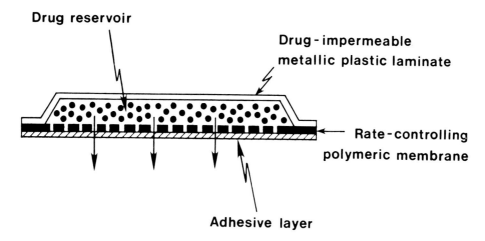

FIGURE 6.   The cross-sectional view of a membrane-moderated transdermal drug delivery system, showing various major structural components.

Table 1
TRANSDERM-NITRO® SYSTEM: COMPONENT PROPERTIES[11]

	Component		
	Silicone adhesive	Membrane	Drug reservoir[a]
Fraction of loading dose (% w/w)	8.0	—	92.0
Nitroglycerin solubility (mg/ml)	50.0	6.0	2.0
Thickness (μm)	30.0	50.0	—
Diffusion coefficient (cm²/hr × 10⁴)	6.0	0.456	144.0

[a]   One gram of drug reservoir is contained in every 20 cm² device.

$$P_m = \frac{K_{m/r} \cdot D_m}{h_m} \tag{6}$$

$$P_a = \frac{K_{a/m} \cdot D_a}{h_a} \tag{7}$$

where $K_{m/r}$ and $K_{a/m}$ are the partition coefficient for the interfacial partitioning of drug from the reservoir to the membrane and from the membrane to the adhesive, respectively; D_m and D_a are the diffusion coefficient in the rate-controlling membrane and adhesive layer, respectively; h_m and h_a are the thickness of the rate-controlling membrane and adhesive layer, respectively. In the case of microporous membrane, the porosity and tortuosity factors of the membrane should be taken into calculation of the D_m and h_m values. Substituting Equations 6 and 7 for P_m and P_a in Equation 5 gives

$$\frac{dQ}{dt} = \frac{K_{m/r}K_{a/m} \cdot D_a \cdot C_R}{K_{m/r}D_m h_a + K_{a/m}D_a h_m} \tag{8}$$

ADHESIVE DIFFUSION-CONTROLLED

TRANSDERMAL DRUG DELIVERY SYSTEMS

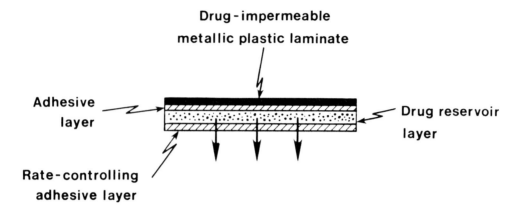

FIGURE 7.   The cross-sectional view of an adhesive diffusion-controlled transdermal drug delivery system, showing various major structural components.

which defines the intrinsic rate of drug release from a membrane-moderated drug delivery system described here.

The membrane permeation-controlled transdermal drug delivery has also been applied to the development of transdermal therapeutic systems for the controlled percutaneous absorption of estradiol,[15,16] clonidine,[17] nitroglycerin,[18] and prostaglandin derivative.[19]

B. Adhesive Diffusion-Controlled Transdermal Drug Delivery Systems

This type of drug delivery system is a simplified version of the membrane-moderated drug delivery system described earlier in the first approach. Instead of completely encapsulating the drug reservoir in a compartment fabricated from a drug-impermeable metallic plastic backing, the drug reservoir is formulated by directly dispersing the drug in an adhesive polymer and then spreading the medicated adhesive by solvent casting onto a flat sheet of drug-impermeable metallic plastic backing to form a thin drug reservoir layer (Figure 7). On the top of the drug reservoir layer, layers of nonmedicated, rate-controlling adhesive polymer of constant thickness are spread to produce an adhesive diffusion-controlled drug delivery system. The rate of drug release is defined by:

$$\frac{dQ}{dt} = \frac{K_{a/r} \cdot D_a \cdot C_R}{h_a} \tag{9}$$

where $K_{a/r}$ is the partition coefficient for the interfacial partitioning of drug from the reservoir layer to the adhesive layer.

This type of transdermal drug delivery system is best illustrated by the development and marketing of Deponit® system (Pharma-Schwartz GmbH, Monheim, Germany) in Europe for one-a-day medication of angina pectoris. This adhesive diffusion-controlled drug delivery system is also applied to the transdermal controlled administration of verapamil.

C. Matrix Dispersion-Type Transdermal Drug Delivery Systems

In this approach, the drug reservoir is formed by homogeneously dispersing the drug solids in a hydrophilic or lipophilic polymer matrix and the medicated polymer is then molded into a medicated disc with a defined surface area and controlled thickness. This

MATRIX DISPERSION-TYPE

TRANSDERMAL DRUG DELIVERY SYSTEMS

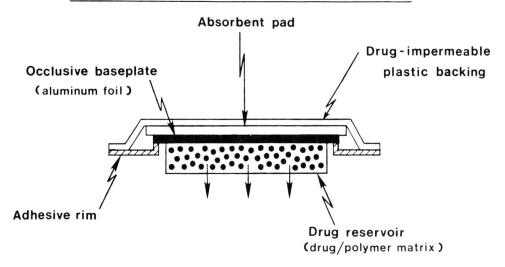

FIGURE 8.   The cross-sectional view of a matrix dispersion-type transdermal drug delivery system, showing various major structural components.

drug reservoir-containing polymer disc is then glued onto an occlusive baseplate in a compartment fabricated from a drug-impermeable plastic backing (Figure 8). Instead of spreading the adhesive polymer onto the surface of the medicated disc as discussed earlier in the first two approaches, the adhesive polymer is applied along the circumference to form a strip of adhesive rim around the medicated disc. The rate of drug release from this matrix dispersion-type drug delivery system is defined as:

$$\frac{dQ}{dt} = \left(\frac{ACpDp}{2t}\right)^{1/2} \tag{10}$$

where A is the initial drug loading dose dispersed in the polymer matrix; Cp and Dp are the solubility and diffusivity of the drug in the polymer, respectively. In view of the fact that only the drug species dissolved in the polymer can release, so Cp is essentially equal to C_R.

At steady state, a Q *vs.* $t^{1/2}$ drug release profile is obtained as defined by:

$$\frac{Q}{t^{1/2}} = [(2A - Cp)CpDp]^{1/2} \tag{11}$$

This type of transdermal drug delivery system is exemplified by the development of Nitro-Dur® system[20] (Key Pharmaceuticals, Inc., Miami, Fla.), which has been approved by FDA for one-a-day medication of angina pectoris. Patent disclosures have also been filed for applying this drug delivery system for transdermal controlled administration of estradiol diacetate and verapamil.

D. Microreservoir-Type Transdermal Drug Delivery Systems

This type of drug delivery system can be considered as the hybrid of reservoir and matrix dispersion-type drug delivery systems. In this approach, the drug reservoir is formed by

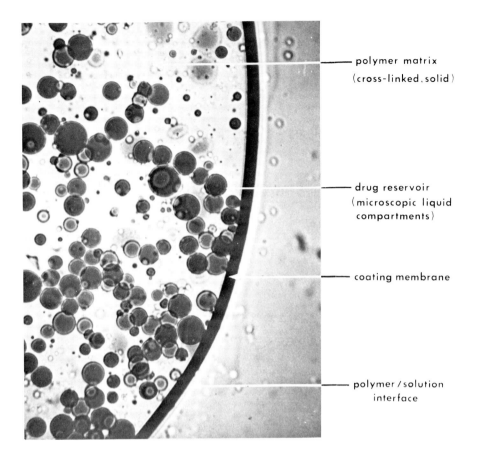

FIGURE 9.   Photomicrograph of a microreservoir-type drug delivery system, showing the microscopic structure of the system.

suspending the drug solids in an aqueous solution of water-soluble liquid polymer. The drug suspension is then dispersed homogeneously in a lipophilic polymer, by high-shear mechanical force, to form thousands of unleachable, microscopic spheres of drug reservoirs. This thermodynamically unstable dispersion is stabilized by immediately cross-linking the polymer chains *in situ* (Figure 9), which produces a medicated polymer disc with a constant surface area and a fixed thickness. A transdermal therapeutic system thus formed with the medicated disc positioned at the center and surrounded by an adhesive rim (Figure 10). This technology has been utilized in the development and marketing of Nitrodisc® system (Searle Pharmaceuticals, Inc., Chicago, Ill.) for one-a-day treatment of angina pectoris.[9,21-24]

The rate of drug release from the microsealed drug delivery system is defined by:

$$\frac{dQ}{dt} = \frac{D_p D_s \alpha' K_p}{D_p h_d + D_s h_p \alpha' K_p} \left[\beta S_p - \frac{D_l S_l (1 - \beta)}{h_l} \left(\frac{1}{K_l} + \frac{1}{K_m} \right) \right] \qquad (12)$$

where $\alpha' = \partial'/\beta'$. ∂' is the ratio of drug concentration in the bulk of elution solution over drug solubility in the elution solution and β' is the ratio of drug concentration at the outer edge of the polymer coating membrane over drug solubility in the polymer coating membrane; K_l, K_m, and K_p are the partition coefficients for the interfacial partitioning of drug from the liquid compartment to the polymer matrix, from the polymer matrix to the polymer coating membrane, and from the polymer coating membrane to the elution solution (or skin), re-

MICRORESERVOIR-TYPE

TRANSDERMAL DRUG DELIVERY SYSTEMS

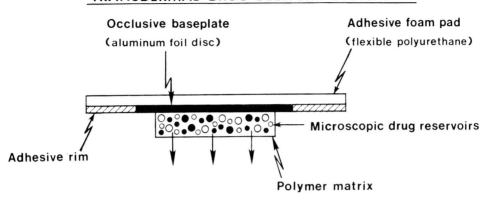

FIGURE 10.   The cross-sectional view of a microreservoir-type transdermal drug delivery system, showing various major structural components.

spectively; D_l, D_p, and D_s are the diffusivities of the drug in the liquid compartment, polymer coating membrane, and elution solution (or skin), respectively: S_l and S_p are the solubilities of the drug in the liquid compartment and in the polymer matrix, respectively; h_l, h_p, and h_d are the thicknesses of the liquid layer surrounding the drug particles, the polymer coating membrane around the polymer matrix, and the hydrodynamic diffusion layer surrounding the polymer coating membrane, respectively; β is the ratio of drug concentration at the inner edge of the interfacial barrier over the drug solubility in the polymer matrix.

Release of drugs from the microreservoir-type drug delivery system can follow a partition-control of matrix diffusion-control process depending upon the relative magnitude of S_l and S_p.[25] The resulting release follows a *Q. vs. t* or *Q. vs. $t^{1/2}$* profile, respectively. For the nitroglycerin system, a matrix diffusion-control process is obtained.

Other types of drug delivery systems are also under investigation for possible applications in the transdermal controlled administration of drugs. It is exemplified by the development of a Poroplastic® membrane[26] and a hydrophilic polymeric reservoir.[27] Both of them are drug solution-saturated porous polymer matrices.

IV. KINETIC EVALUATIONS OF TRANSDERMAL DRUG DELIVERY SYSTEMS

The release and skin permeation kinetics of drug from these four technologically different transdermal therapeutic systems can be evaluated using a diffusion cell under identical conditions. It can be carried out by mounting, individually, the full-thickness abdominal skin, which has been freshly excised from human cadaver or hairless mouse,[29] on an 8-cell Franz diffusion assembly (Figure 4). The drug delivery systems are then applied with their drug-releasing surface in intimate contact with the stratum corneum surface of the skin. The skin permeation profile of drug is followed by sampling the receptor solution at predetermined intervals for a duration of up to 30 hr and assaying drug concentrations in the samples by a sensitive analytical method, such as high performance liquid chromatography (HPLC) method.[10] The release profiles of drug from these transdermal therapeutic systems can also be investigated using the same experimental setup without the skin.[10]

A. In Vitro Drug Release Kinetics

Using nitroglycerin as the example, the controlled release of drugs from these four tech-

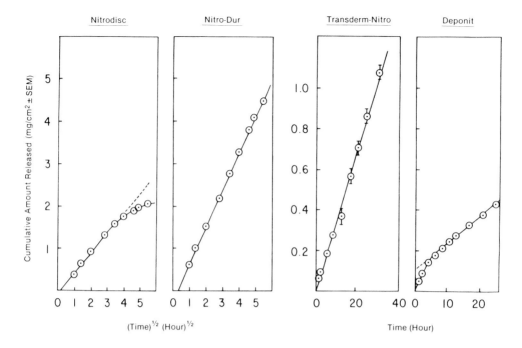

FIGURE 11.   Comparative release profiles of nitroglycerin from various transdermal drug delivery systems into saline solution containing 20% PEG 400 at 37°C. The release flux of nitroglycerin is Nitrodisc® system (2.443 ± 0.136 mg/cm²/day$^{1/2}$), Nitro-Dur® system (4.124 ± 0.047 mg/cm²/day$^{1/2}$), Transderm-Nitro® system (0.843 ± 0.035 mg/cm²/day), Deponit system (0.324 ± 0.011 mg/cm²/day).[10]

nologically different transdermal therapeutic systems can be illustrated and compared. The results indicated that nitroglycerin is released at a constant rate profile (*Q vs. t*) from the Transderm-Nitro® system (a membrane-moderated transdermal drug delivery system) and the Deponit system (an adhesive diffusion-controlled transdermal drug delivery system) (Figure 11). The release rate of nitroglycerin from the Transderm-Nitro® system (0.843 ± 0.035 mg/cm²/day) is almost three times greater than that from the Deponit system (0.324 ± 0.011 mg/cm²/day).

On the other hand, the release profiles of nitroglycerin from Nitrodisc® and Nitro-Dur® systems are not constant, but are observed to follow a linear *Q. vs. t*$^{1/2}$ relationship as expected from the matrix diffusion-controlled drug release kinetics.[30] The release flux of nitroglycerin from the Nitro-Dur® system (a matrix dispersion-type transdermal drug delivery system) is about twice that from the Nitrodisc® system (a microreservoir-type transdermal drug delivery system) (4.124 ± 0.047 vs. 2.443 ± 0.136 mg/cm²/day$^{1/2}$). Apparently, the mechanisms and rates of nitroglycerin release from these four drug delivery systems are quite different from one another, as expected from Equations 8, 9, 11, and 12.

B. In Vitro Skin Permeation Kinetics — Animal Model

Interestingly, the skin permeation studies through hairless mouse skin suggested that all four transdermal therapeutic systems provide a constant rate of skin permeation as expected from Equation 3 (Figure 12). A highest rate of skin permeation was observed with the Nitrodisc® system (0.426 ± 0.024 mg/cm²/day), but only one of the systems is statistically no different from the rate of skin permeation for pure nitroglycerin (0.476 ± 0.041 mg/cm²/day, Figure 5). For the Nitro-Dur® system, practically the same rate of skin permeation (0.408 ± 0.024 mg/cm²/day) was observed initially and 12 hr later, however, the rate was slowed down to 0.248 (±0.018) mg/cm²/day. On the other hand, the rate of skin permeation

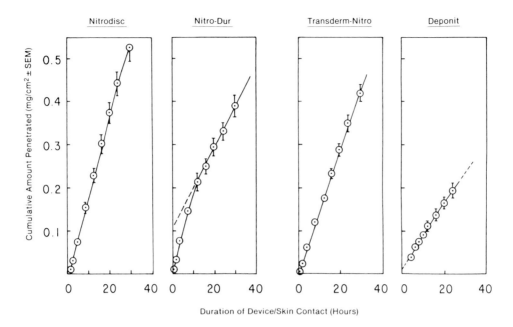

FIGURE 12. Comparative permeation profiles of nitroglycerin from various transdermal drug delivery systems through the hairless mouse abdominal skin at 37°C. The rate of skin permeation is Nitrodisc® system (0.426 ± 0.024 mg/cm²/day), Nitro-Dur® system [0.408 ± 0.024 mg/cm²/day (<12 hr)]; [0.248 ± 0.018 mg/cm²/day (>12 hr)], Transderm-Nitro® system (0.338 ± 0.017 mg/cm²/day), Deponit system (0.175 ± 0.016 mg/cm²/day).[10]

of nitroglycerin delivered by the Transderm-Nitro® system (0.338 ± 0.017 mg/cm²/day) was found to be 30% lower than the rate achieved by pure nitroglycerin (0.476 mg/cm²/day). The lowest rate of skin permeation was observed with Deponit system (0.175 ± 0.016 mg/cm²/day), which is only 37% of the skin permeation rate for pure nitroglycerin through hairless mouse skin. The relevance of these differences for hairless mouse skin should be questioned, since at least three of the commercial systems have equivalent bioavailability to nitroglycerin ointment.

Comparing the rate of skin permeation with the rate of release indicated that under the sink conditions all transdermal therapeutic systems release nitroglycerin at a rate which is greater than the rate of uptake by the skin, i.e., $R_r \gg R_a$ (Figure 2). For example, nitroglycerin was released from Transderm-Nitro® system, which is a membrane permeation-controlled drug delivery system, at a rate (0.843 mg/cm²/day) which is 2.5 times greater than the rate of uptake by the skin (0.338 mg/cm²/day). Likewise, the rate of release from the Deponit system, which is an adhesive diffusion-controlled drug delivery system and releases nitroglycerin at the slowest rate (Figure 11), was also 1.9-fold faster than the rate of skin permeation (0.324 vs. 0.175 mg/cm²/day). The same observations were also true for Nitrodisc® and Nitro-Dur® systems. This phenomenon is indicative of the rate-limiting role of stratum corneum in the skin permeation of drugs as a result of its low permeability.

C. In Vitro Skin Permeation Kinetics — Human Cadaver

The permeation of nitroglycerin across the human cadaver skin was also investigated for the Transderm-Nitro® system, the membrane permeation-controlled transdermal drug delivery system, and for the Nitro-Dur® system, the matrix diffusion-controlled transdermal drug delivery system.[31] The results (Figure 13) indicated that the skin permeation of nitroglycerin through the human cadaver abdominal epidermis also follows the same zero-order kinetic profile as observed with hairless mouse abdominal skin (Figure 12). It is interesting to note that the rates of skin permeation generated from the excised skins of hairless mouse and

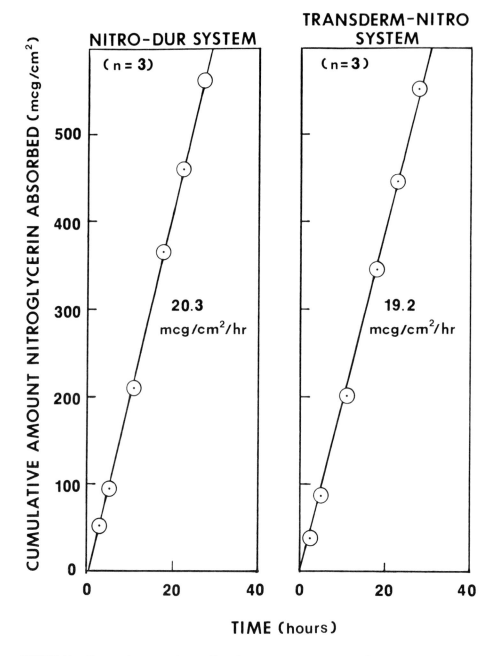

FIGURE 13.   Comparative permeation profiles of nitroglycerin from Nitro-Dur® and Transderm-Nitro® systems across the human cadaver abdominal epidermis. The rate of skin permeation is Nitro-Dur® system (20.3 µg/cm²/hr) and Transderm-Nitro® system (19.2 µg/cm²/hr).[29]

human cadaver are in fairly good agreement (Table 2), suggesting that hairless mouse skin could be an acceptable animal model for human skin in the skin permeation studies of nitroglycerin.

D. In Vivo Transdermal Bioavailability in Humans

The transdermal bioavailability of nitroglycerin resulted from the 24- to 32-hr topical applications of various transdermal therapeutic systems in human volunteers, as indicated

Table 2
IN VITRO-IN VIVO COMPARISON ON SKIN
PERMEATION RATES OF NITROGLYCERIN

| | Skin permeation rates (mg/cm²/day) | | |
| | In vitro | | |
Delivery systems	Hairless mouse	Human cadaver	In vivo[d]
Nitroglycerin alone	0.476[a]	0.312[b]	—
Nitrodisc®	0.426	—	0.473
Nitro-Dur®	0.408	0.487[c]	0.412
Transderm-Nitro®	0.338	0.461[c]	0.428
Deponit	0.175	—	—

[a] Determined from skin permeation studies of pure nitroglycerin across full-thickness hairless mouse abdominal skin at 37°C.
[b] Determined from an aqueous solution of nitroglycerin at 30°C.[35]
[c] Determined from skin permeation studies at 37°C using the epidermis isolated from human cadaver abdominal skin.[31]
[d] Calculated from Equation 13, in which $k_c = 0.1575/min$ and $V_d = 179.6$ ℓ.[34]

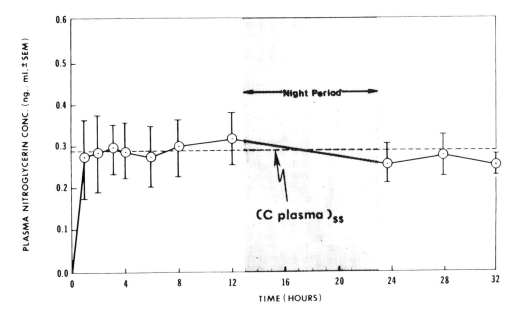

FIGURE 14.   Plasma profiles of nitroglycerin in 12 healthy male volunteers, each received a unit of Nitrodisc® system (16 cm²) on the chest for 32 hr. A steady-state plasma level, (Cp)ss, of 280.6 ± 18.7 pg/mℓ was determined.[24]

by the levels of plasma nitroglycerin, is shown in Figures 14 to 16. Results suggested that a prolonged, steady-state plasma level of nitroglycerin can be achieved and maintained for a duration of at least 24 hr by controlled drug delivery through the transdermal therapeutic systems.

The plasma level was found to be linearly proportional to the drug releasing surface of transdermal therapeutic systems in contact with the skin (Figure 17). For every cm² of the drug releasing surface applied, a plasma level of 14 pg/mℓ was achieved.

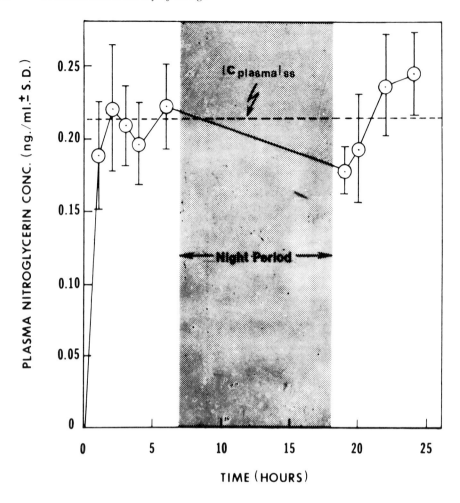

FIGURE 15.   Plasma profiles of nitroglycerin in 14 healthy human subjects, each received a unit of Transderm-Nitro® system (20 cm²) for 24 hr. A (Cp)ss value of 209.8 ± 22.8 pg/mℓ was determined.[12]

E. In Vitro-In Vivo Correlations

To further examine the feasibility of using freshly excised, hairless mouse skin as the animal model for the skin permeation kinetics studies of drug across the human skin, the in vivo rate of skin permeation $(Q/t)_{i.v.}$ should be determined for comparison. It can be calculated, from the steady-state plasma level $(C_p)_{ss}$ data (Figures 14 to 16), according to the following relationship:[32]

$$\left(\frac{Q}{t}\right)_{i.v.} = (C_p)_{ss} \cdot K_e \cdot V_d \tag{13}$$

where K_e is the first-order rate constant for the elimination of drug and V_d is the apparent volume of distribution of drug.

Results indicated that the in vivo skin permeation rates calculated on the basis of Equation 13 show a reasonably good agreement with the in vitro data determined from either human cadaver or hairless mouse skin (Table 2). This in vivo-in vitro agreement provides additional evidence that hairless mouse skin could be an acceptable animal model for studying the skin permeation kinetics of systemically effective drugs, like nitroglycerin, in humans.

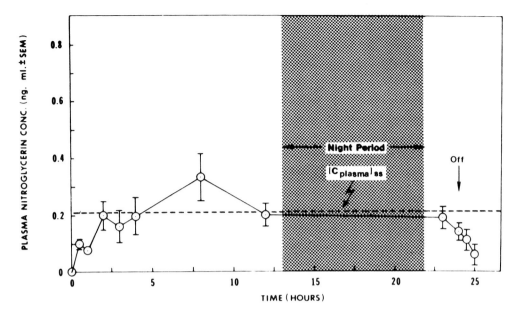

FIGURE 16.   Plasma profiles of nitroglycerin in six normal male volunteers, each received a unit of Nitro-Dur® system (20 cm²) over the chest for 24 hr. A (Cp)ss value of 201.4 ± 60.7 pg/mℓ was determined.[36]

V. FORMULATION DESIGN AND OPTIMIZATION

To formulate a transdermal therapeutic system one should take into consideration the relationship between the rate of drug delivery to the skin surface and the maximum achievable rate of drug absorption by the skin tissue. It is particularly important since the stratum corneum is known to be highly impermeable to many drugs. Perhaps, an ideally designed transdermal therapeutic system should have a rate of drug delivery to the skin surface, so the transdermal bioavailability of a drug becomes independent of any possible intra- and/or interpatient variability in skin permeability. However, if the device controlled the delivery rate, larger surface area patches with poor aesthetics would be required to achieve comparable bioavailabilities of nitroglycerin. Ultimately, nitroglycerin patches which can enhance the flux through skin may achieve this optimization.

The rate of skin permeation $(Q/t)_{ss}$ of a drug at steady state for a membrane-controlled system is related to the actual rate of drug delivery from a transdermal therapeutic system $(Q/t)_{tts}$ to the skin surface and the maximum achievable rate of skin absorption $(Q/t)_{m,s}$ as follows:[33]

$$\frac{1}{(Q/t)_{ss}} = \frac{1}{(Q/t)_{tts}} + \frac{1}{(Q/t)_{m,s}} \tag{14}$$

And, the actual rate of drug delivery from a transdermal therapeutic system to the skin surface (which acts as the receptor medium) can thus be determined from:

$$\frac{1}{(Q/t)_{tts}} = \frac{1}{(Q/t)_{ss}} - \frac{1}{(Q/t)_{m,s}} \tag{15}$$

Using the rate of skin permeation from the pure nitroglycerin as the value for $(Q/t)_{m,s}$, the actual delivery rate of nitroglycerin from various marketed transdermal therapeutic systems can be calculated. Results indicate that the rates of delivery from Nitrodisc,® Nitro-

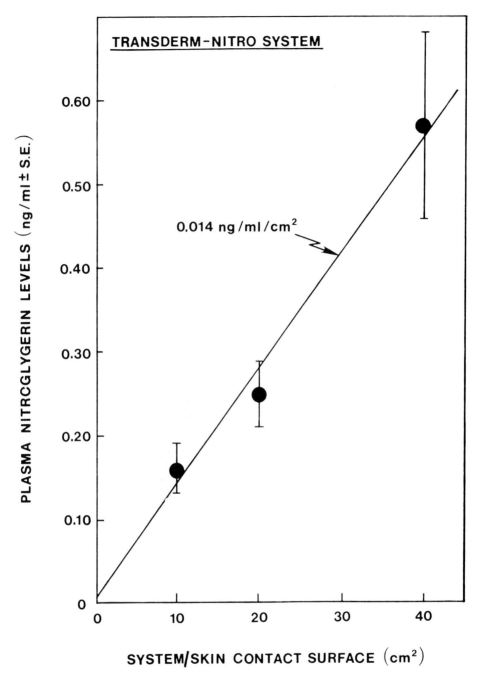

FIGURE 17. Linear relationship between the steady-state plasma nitroglycerin levels in humans and the drug-releasing surface of Transderm-Nitro® system in contact with the skin. A plasma nitroglycerin level of 14 pg/ml was achieved for every cm² of drug-releasing surface applied.[11]

Dur®, and Transderm-Nitro® systems are three to ninefold greater than the maximum achievable rate of skin permeation (0.476 mg/cm²/day) for nitroglycerin: On the other hand, the rate of delivery from Deponit system is only 58% of the maximum rate of skin permeation. In all four systems, the skin serves as a major element for the control of delivery of nitroglycerin.

ACKNOWLEDGMENT

The author wishes to thank Ms. Marline Boslet for her excellent typing of this manuscript.

REFERENCES

1. **Jacob, S. W. and Francone, C. A.,** *Structure and Function of Man,* 2nd ed., W. B. Saunders, Philadelphia, 1970, 55.
2. **Zanowiak, P. and Jacobs, M. R.,** Topical Anti-Infective Products, in *Handbook of Nonprescription Drugs,* 7th ed., Laitin, S. C., Ed., American Pharmaceutical Association, Washington, D.C., 1982, 525.
3. **Chien, Y. W.,** Logics of transdermal controlled drug administration, *Drug Dev. Ind. Pharm.,* 9, 497, 1983.
4. **Kastrup, E. K. and Boyd, J. R.,** *Drug: Facts and Comparisons,* J. B. Lippincott, New York, 1983, 1634.
5. **Shaw, J. E., Bayne, W., and Schmidt, L.,** Clinical pharmacology of scopolamine, *Clin. Pharmacol. Ther.,* 19, 115, 1976.
6. **Armstrong, P. W., Armstrong, J. A., and Marks, G. S.,** Pharmacokinetic-hemodynamic studies of nitroglycerin ointment in congestive heart failure, *Am. J. Cardiol.,* 46, 670, 1980.
7. **Sitruk-Ware, R., deLignieres, B., Basdevant, A., and Mauvais-Jarvis, P.,** Absorption of percutaneous oestradiol in postmenopausal women, *Maturitas,* 2, 207, 1980.
8. **Chien, Y. W.,** *Novel Drug Delivery Systems,* Marcel Dekker, New York, 1982, 149.
9. **Sanvordeker, D. R., Cooney, J. G., and Wester, R. C.,** Transdermal Nitroglycerin Pad, U.S. Patent 4,336,243, 1982.
10. **Keshary, P. R., Huang, Y. C. and Chien, Y. W.,** personal communication, 1984.
11. **Good, W. R.,** Transderm-Nitro®: controlled delivery of nitroglycerin via the transdermal route, *Drug Dev. Ind. Pharm.,* 9, 647, 1983.
12. **Gerardin, A., Hirtz, J., Fankhauser, P., and Moppert, J.,** Achievement of sustained plasma concentrations of nitroglycerin (TNG) in man by a transdermal therapeutic system, in APhA/APS 31st National Meeting Abstracts, Washington, D.C., 11(2), 84, 1981.
13. **Shaw, J. E. and Chandrasekaran, S. K.,** Controlled topical delivery of drugs for systemic action, *Drug Metab. Rev.,* 8, 223, 1978.
14. **Hwang, S., Owada, E., Suhardja, L., Ho, N. F. H., Flynn, G. L., and Higuchi, W. I.,** Systems approach to vaginal delivery of drugs. V. *In situ* vaginal absorption of 1-Alkanoic acids, *J. Pharm. Sci.,* 66, 781, 1977.
15. **Schenkel, L., Balestra, J., Schmitt, L., and Shaw, J.,** Transdermal oestrogen substitution in the menopause, in 2nd Int. Conf. on Drug Absorption — Rate Control in Drug Therapy, Edinburgh, Scotland, 1983, 41.
16. **Laufer, L. R., De Fazio, J. L., Lu, J. K. H., Meldrum, D. R., Eggena, P., Sambhi, M. P., Hershman, J. M., and Judd, H. L.,** Estrogen replacement therapy by transdermal estradiol administration, *Am. J. Obstet. Gynecol.,* 146, 533, 1983.
17. **Arndts, D. and Arndts, K.,** Pharmacokinetics and pharmacodynamics of transdermally administered clonidine, *Eur. J. Clin. Pharmacol.,* 26, 79, 1984.
18. **Kydonieus, A. F., Kauffman, D., Lambert, C., Berner, B., Lambert, H., Geising, D., Frazier, W., Morris, R., and Niebergall, P.,** Transdermal delivery of nitroglycerin from a laminated reservoir system, in Proc. of 11th Int. Symp. on Controlled Release Bioactive Materials, Meyers, W. E. and Dunn, R. L., Eds., Ft. Lauderdale, Fla., 1984, 32.
19. **Roseman, T. J., Bennett, R. M., Biermacher, J. J., Tuttle, M. E., and Spilman, C. H.,** Design criteria for carbopost methyl controlled release devices, in Proc. of 11th Int. Symp. on Controlled Release Bioactive Materials, Meyers, W. E. and Dunn, R. L., Eds., Ft. Lauderdale, Fla., 1984, 50.
20. **Keith, A. D.,** Polymer matrix considerations for transdermal devices, *Drug Dev. Ind. Pharm.,* 9, 605, 1983.
21. **Chien, Y. W. and Lambert, H. J.,** Microsealed Pharmaceutical Delivery Devices, U.S. Patent 3,946,106, 1976.
22. **Chien, Y. W. and Lambert, H. J.,** Method for Making a Microsealed Delivery Device, U.S. Patent 3,992,518, 1976.
23. **Chien, Y. W. and Lambert, H. J.,** Microsealed Pharmaceutical Delivery Device, U.S. Patent 4,053,580, 1977.

24. **Karim, A.,** Transdermal absorption: a unique opportunity for constant delivery of nitroglycerin, *Drug Dev. Ind. Pharm.,* 9, 671, 1983.
25. **Chien, Y. W.,** Microsealed drug delivery systems: theoretical aspects and biomedical assessments, in *Int. Symp. on Recent Advances in Drug Delivery Systems,* Anderson, J. M. and Kim, S. W., Eds., Plenum Press, New York, 1984, 367.
26. **Davidson, S. J., Nichols, L. D., Obermayer, A. S., Allen, M. B., Murphy, E. J., and Hurd, R. N.,** Developing a Controlled Release Dual-Antibiotic Wound Dressing, in Proc. of 11th Int. Symp. on Controlled Release Bioactive Materials, Meyers, W. E. and Dunn, R. L., Eds., Ft. Lauderdale, Fla., 1984, 58.
27. **Hymes, A. C.,** A hydrophilic polymeric reservoir for transdermal drug delivery, in AphA/APS Midwest Regional Meeting Abstract, Chicago, April, 1984, 4.
28. **Chien, Y. W.,** Long-term, navel controlled administration of testosterone, *J. Pharm. Sci.,* (in press).
29. **Durrheim, H., Flynn, G. L., Higuchi, W. I., and Behl, C. R.,** Permeation of hairless mouse skin. I. Experimental methods and comparison with human epidermal permeation by alkanols, *J. Pharm. Sci.,* 69, 781, 1980.
30. **Chien, Y. W.,** *Novel Drug Delivery Systems,* Marcel Dekker, New York, 1982, 465.
31. **Magnuson, D. E.,** personal communication, 1983.
32. **Chien, Y. W.,** Pharmaceutical considerations of transdermal nitroglycerin delivery: the various approaches, *Am. Heart J.,* 108, 207, 1984.
33. **Shaw, J. E., Chandrasekaran, S. K., Michaels, A. S., and Taskovich, L.,** Controlled transdermal delivery, in vitro and in vivo, in *Animal Models in Dermatology,* Maibach, H., Ed., Churchill Livingston, Edinburgh, 1975, chap. 14.
34. **Armstrong, P. W., Armstrong, J. A., and Marks, G. S.,** Blood levels after sublingual nitroglycerin, *Circulation,* 59, 585, 1979.
35. **Michaels, A. S., Chandrasekaran, S. K., and Shaw, J. E.,** Drug permeation through human skin: theory and in vitro experimental measurement, *A.I.Ch.E. J.,* 21, 985, 1975.
36. **Keith, A. D.,** personal communication, 1983.

Chapter 8

RATE-CONTROLLED TRANSDERMAL THERAPY UTILIZING POLYMERIC MEMBRANES

Jane E. Shaw, Marilou Powers Cramer, and Robert Gale

TABLE OF CONTENTS

I. INTRODUCTION

In the late 1970s, technology became available to permit reproducible, reliable drug administration through intact skin.[1,2] Utilizing dense or porous membranes as the controlling element, compact multicomponent dosage forms solved, in part, several problems that had impeded transdermal therapy, including imprecision of dosing and inconvenient regimens and dosage forms. The latter were principally creams or ointments that required multiple daily applications and were difficult to apply to skin uniformly. Thus, attaining and maintaining predictable drug concentrations in plasma (Figures 1 and 2) was not possible, and transdermal therapy was confined to agents having a wide therapeutic window.

Introduction of rate-controlled systems expanded the advantages of transdermal treatment to include the following:

- Precise control over drug concentrations in plasma to permit increased selectivity of drug actions (i.e., maintained efficacy with reduced side effects). Thus, potent agents with a narrow range in effective plasma concentrations became suitable for administration through skin.
- Multiday continuous drug delivery at a virtually constant rate during wearing of a transdermal dosage form. That capability permitted feasible regimens for very short half-life drugs, and enhanced regimens for others.
- More predictable systemic drug input. Avoidance of the oral route prevents such known variables of the gastrointestinal tract as pH, food content, and motility from unpredictably affecting drug absorption.
- Reduced daily amounts of drug effective through avoidance of first-pass hepatic metabolism. That avoidance also reduces hepatotoxic hazards.
- An external dosage form that is simply and easily removed in case of need to discontinue therapy.
- A noninvasive parenteral route free of the hazards and inconvenience of intramuscular injections or intravenous infusions.

Transdermal dosage forms lacking a rate-controlling element provide some of the advantages listed above but cannot precisely control or maintain drug levels in blood. Control confers important increments in the safety, efficacy, reliability, and acceptability of drug treatment (Table 1).

Any projected development of a transdermal dosage form must take into consideration the physicochemical, pharmacokinetic, and pharmacodynamic properties of the drug. Not all the above-mentioned advantages may be attainable — or needed — for any one drug. Moreover, most drugs do not permeate skin at sufficient rates to be administered from patches of reasonable size. At this time, only potent drugs free of serious irritating or allergenic effects are suitable for transdermal therapy, and only drugs presenting substantial therapeutic disadvantages in their conventional forms justify the expense of transdermal dosage form development.

Yet, when all these exclusions are made, there remains an impressive number of important drugs whose use effectiveness could be improved by controlled delivery through intact skin. Moreover, the number of drugs qualifying for transdermal administration will undoubtedly increase. This increase should partially stem from advances in delivery technology and incorporation of new chemical entities into transdermal dosage forms.

II. MAINTENANCE OF TARGETED DRUG CONCENTRATIONS

Maintenance of a specific drug concentration in blood requires more than simply providing

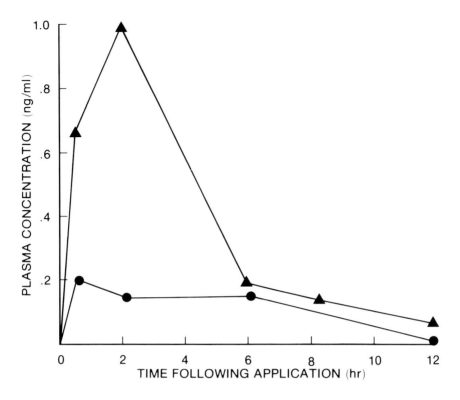

FIGURE 1. Differing plasma concentrations of nitroglycerin in two subjects following topical application of 2% nitroglycerin ointment over 10 cm^2 of skin.

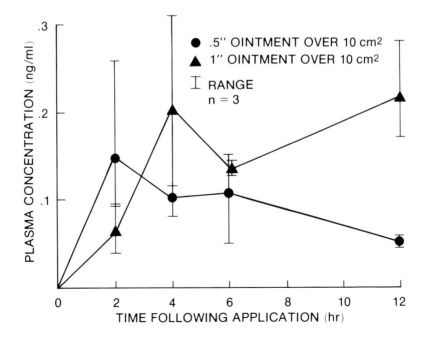

FIGURE 2. Mean plasma concentration of nitroglycerin following application of 0.5 or 1 in. of 2% nitroglycerin ointment over 10 cm^2 of skin.

Table 1

ADVANTAGES[a] OF TRANSDERMAL RATE-CONTROLLED DRUG DELIVERY

	Precision of systemic drug input	Multiday, continuous drug delivery	Avoidance of GI tract and first pass through liver	Noninvasive parenteral route	External dosage form
Safety/efficacy advantages	Maintenance of steady, nontoxic, effective concentrations of drug in plasma	Consistency of therapy over prolonged dosage interval — up to 7 days — great advantage in chronic disease	Lower doses often effective Hepatic toxicity lessened	Infection or extravasation hazards lessened or eliminated	Easily retrievable if termination of treatment is necessary
Acceptability for patient	More comfortable therapy	Convenient undemanding regimen	No gastric discomfort	Convenient, and painless, unlike infusion or infection	Patients often prefer it to oral or i.m. dosing
Reliability	Dosage form controls systemic drug input, rather than the individually varying barrier properties of skin	Patient compliance encouraged	Drug absorption not affected by variables of GI tract or hepatic metabolism	Avoidance of errors or delays in administering i.v. or i.m. medication	Visibility makes presence (and continuity of therapy) easy to check

[a] Not all advantages available (or needed) with any one drug or system.

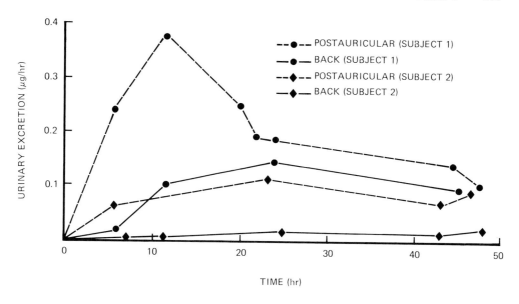

FIGURE 3.   Urinary excretion of scopolamine free base during use of a scopolamine transdermal system (effective area 0.71 cm^2).

controlled release of drug from the dosage form. Two other factors affect drug concentrations in plasma, permeability of the skin to the drug and drug clearance rates — which can both show wide variations among individuals (Figure 3). To assure desired plasma concentrations, these individual differences must be minimized. Clearance differences can be accommodated by providing transdermal dosage forms of different strengths (drug release rates) such that the physician can titrate the patient to the appropriate strength. Negating skin permeability differences requires vesting major control over systemic drug input in the dosage form rather than skin.

That objective can be accomplished to varying degrees by designing the dosage form so that its resistance to drug flow is greater than that of the epidermis (the major locus of the barrier properties of the skin). If all the resistance were in the dosage form, then it would have 100% control over systemic drug input; that is, the rate of drug release to the systemic circulation would equal the drug release rate from the dosage form.

In practice, this has been approached by delivery of the drug from the dosage form at a rate that is below the rate at which the drug can permeate even the most impermeable skin. The obverse situation, where the drug is released much faster than the skin can accept it, makes the variable barrier properties of skin the determinant of the systemic dosage. In such a situation patients with highly permeable skin will absorb much larger doses than others. Thus, for drugs with a narrow therapeutic window, a high degree of control must be vested in the system.

The four membrane-control systems described here provide varying degrees of control over systemic drug dosage, and different durations of drug delivery. It is appropriate to examine their similarities and differences in light of the advantages sought and attained during their development.

III. FOUR TRANSDERMAL SYSTEMS: SIMILARITIES AND DIFFERENCES

The four dosage forms — for rate-controlled delivery of scopolamine, nitroglycerin, clonidine, and estradiol — all contain a backing membrane, drug reservoir, rate-controlling element, adhesive, and a protective release liner that is removed before use. In addition, the systems all incorporate priming doses of drug in the contact adhesive; these doses expedite the achievement of therapeutic drug levels in plasma by satisfying drug solubility and binding sites in the epidermis, as well as the volume of distribution. Thereafter, the slower, steady rate of drug release from the reservoir through the membrane maintains the required plasma levels, providing a full therapeutic effect.

These four dosage forms are representative of the rate-controlled systems so far developed. Despite their common features, however, none can be described as generic. That is, none provides a template for the development of a therapeutic system for another drug. Too many variables, pertaining to each drug — its permeation properties, effective parenteral dose, potential for inducing sensitivity, potency, therapeutic window, half-life, clearance, etc. — must be explored in designing the rate-controlled transdermal dosage form.[3]

Indeed, the four systems have as many differences as similarities. The composition of each differs, and at least two methods of manufacture are used. The scopolamine and clonidine dosage forms are multilaminates, which use technologies available in the adhesive and coating industries.[4]

Drug and adhesive layers of these multilaminate systems are prepared by dissolving adhesive polymers in an appropriate vehicle and then adding a drug to each solution. These solutions are then deposited as a thin continuous film onto a moving web that passes through a series of drying ovens. When dried, the drug and adhesive layers, along with the release liner, control membrane, and backing layer, are laminated together. The film laminate is passed through a rotary die cutting press where individual dosage forms are cut. The transdermal systems are then packaged.

The nitroglycerin and estradiol systems are based on form, fill, and seal technology. That is, the drug reservoir is filled as a semisolid or liquid between the backing and rate-controlling membrane, instead of being incorporated in a polymeric layer.

The nitroglycerin, clonidine, and estradiol systems have been developed with a range of drug release rates. These rates are directly proportional to the areas of the systems.

IV. TRANSDERMAL SCOPOLAMINE ADMINISTRATION

Scopolamine, like other antimuscarinic drugs, has many potentially useful pharmacologic actions that currently are underutilized. Of this class of agents, Weiner[5] states that the agents "have been employed in a wide variety of clinical conditions . . . However, the lack of selectivity . . . makes it difficult to obtain desired therapeutic responses without concomitant side effects. The latter usually are not serious but are sufficiently disturbing to the patient to limit sharply the dosage tolerated and therefore the usefulness of these agents, particularly for chronic administration."

In motion sickness, scopolamine has been considered the most effective drug.[2,6,7] However, central nervous system (CNS) side actions and the need for four to six daily doses have impeded use of this drug. Thus, greater selectivity of action, prolonged effectiveness, and a convenient dosage form were objectives in the development of the transdermal scopolamine dosage form.

Scopolamine is a suitable drug for rate-controlled transdermal delivery. It is nonirritating to skin; it is potent (effective oral or intramuscular (i.m.) dose 200 μg); its actions are concentration-dependent (Figure 4); and its half-life is less than an hour. Continuous delivery of scopolamine at a controlled rate offered the promise of separating desired from undesired effects and making dosage interval independent of drug half-life.

Figure 4 shows the increasing number of pharmacologic responses elicited by rising blood concentrations of scopolamine (reflected by various urinary excretion rates) in volunteers receiving 200 μg i.m. doses. Motion sickness is prevented by blood concentrations in plasma that are lower than those associated with the undesirable CNS effects of the drug. Figure

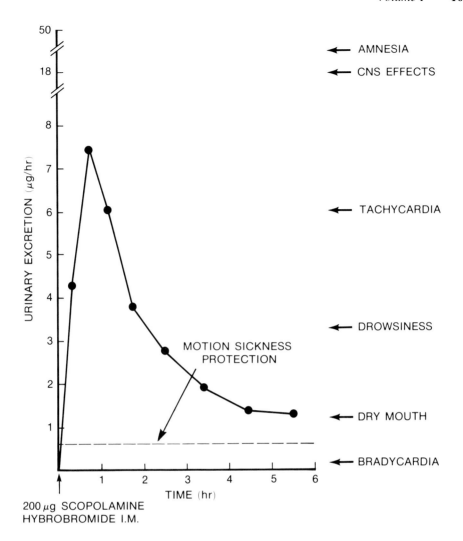

FIGURE 4. Relationship between blood levels of scopolamine (as reflected in amount of drug excreted in urine) and pharmacologic effects.

3, however, demonstrates the difficulty of achieving selectivity of action in all patients simply by controlling release rate from the dosage form. These two subjects, like many others, differ widely in their absorption of the drug through the same skin site — in this instance, the back and postauricular areas. To negate these differences, the drug had to be delivered at a rate far lower than its permeation rate through average skin. Since permeation of drug through the postauricular area is highest (Figure 5), placement there offered the best opportunity to achieve a wide differential between a therapeutic delivery rate from the dosage form and the rate at which the skin could accept it. Although the scopolamine delivery rate selected was only 2 μg/cm²/hr, the drug is so potent that the area had to be only 2.5 cm² to deliver an effective systemic dose. That size is feasible for a patch to be worn behind the ear. The therapeutic dose — only 0.5 mg over 3 days — is one fifth of the oral or i.m. dose usually administered over that time period; yet, it prevented motion sickness in 75% of susceptible subjects in clinical trials.[8] Transient dryness of the mouth was the only significant side effect. In subsequent general use, the incidence of more troublesome side effects has been low, and efficacy high.

This selectivity is attributable to the low transdermal dose and to the lack of peaking drug

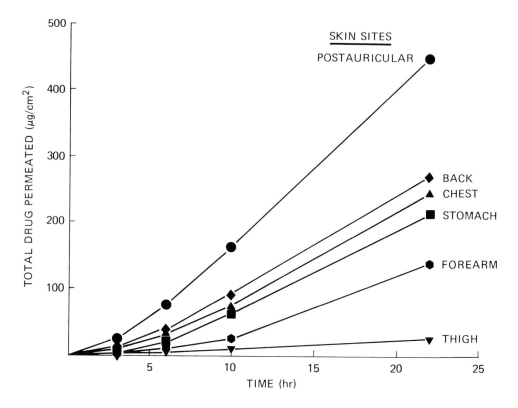

FIGURE 5.   In vitro permeation of scopolamine base through human skin obtained from various body sites.

concentrations in plasma that occur with other dosage forms (Figure 6). Figure 7 demonstrates how precisely the membrane within the system controls scopolamine concentrations in plasma. The concentrations over 72 hr are almost identical to those achieved with a rate-controlled intravenous (i.v.) infusion. That degree of control is highly desirable for a drug with a narrow therapeutic window such as scopolamine. (The 3-day system functionality represents the usual period of time required to become tolerant to motion.)

In summary, it may be said that the first transdermal therapeutic system to reach routine medical use attained the objectives sought, a lessening of parasympatholytic side actions, prolonged efficacy following one application, and suitability for use in the presence of nausea.

Whether these advantages mean that scopolamine will undergo a renaissance for indications other than motion sickness remains to be seen. Its numerous pharmacologic actions favor this possibility. At present, results from preliminary clinical trials suggest its usefulness in vertigo.[9,10]

V. TRANSDERMAL NITROGLYCERIN ADMINISTRATION

The use of nitroglycerin has been limited principally by its extremely short duration of action rather than by its therapeutic window, which is wide. Even with blood concentrations of 3000 ng/mℓ, the principal side effect is a headache to which patients can become tolerant. However, the 3-min half-life of the drug has prevented its widespread use for prevention of angina, as well as its use for other possible cardiovascular indications. Nitrate slow-release oral tablets and nitroglycerin ointments both require dosing several times daily. The ointments — in addition to being inconvenient to apply — do not achieve uniform plasma concentrations (Figure 1).

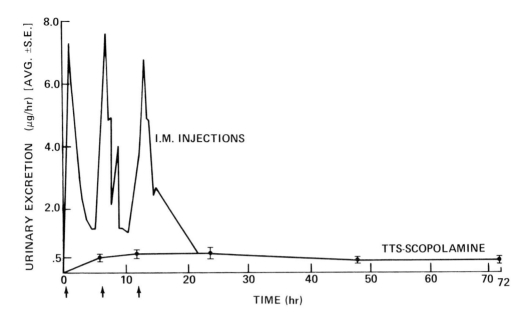

FIGURE 6. Urinary excretion rates following three intramuscular injections of 200 μg scopolamine hydrobromide and during use of the scopolamine transdermal therapeutic system (Transderm® Scōp).

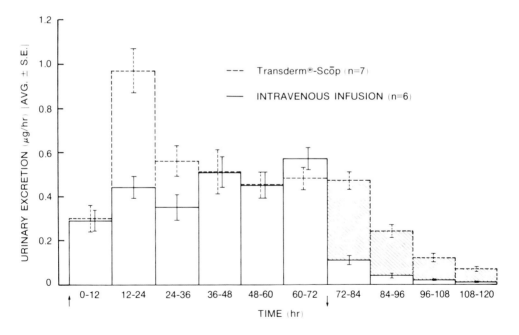

FIGURE 7. Excretion of scopolamine base in urine during and following transdermal (Transderm® Scōp) and rate-controlled intravenous administration. Drug administration started at 0 hr and ended at 72 hr.

Thus, the three aims of developing a membrane-controlled transdermal nitroglycerin dosage form were, in order of importance: prolonged drug efficacy after one application, simplicity of administration, and sufficient control over systemic drug input to prevent dose-dumping. Dose-dumping was expected to be a problem only among patients whose skin permeability was above average. Factors causing individuals to differ in skin permeability include age, sex, race, skin condition, e.g., abrasions, sunburn, disease, as well as transient factors such as changes in body and skin temperature, moisture content, and systemic disease.

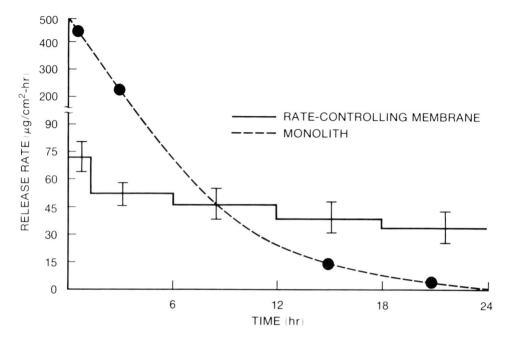

FIGURE 8.   In vitro nitroglycerin release rates from the Transderm®-Nitro and a monolithic system releasing nitroglycerin in dissolution testing.

Studies with monolithic dosage forms indicated that unusually permeable skin itself would not provide a sufficient barrier to prevent overdosing. These dosage forms released the drug at a sharply declining rate in vitro in dissolution testing[11] (Figure 8). While such testing certainly is relevant to the prevention of the overdosing of subjects with unusually permeable skin, the relevance of release in dissolution testing from monoliths to the general subject population is questionable (see, for example, Chapter 9). The in vitro release pattern for monoliths (Figure 8) raised two possibilities, excessive drug input to the systemic circulation at the beginning of the dosage interval for patients with highly permeable skin and inadequate dosage later. Thus, a multicomponent system was designed to exert the needed degree of control over the systemic input rate of the drug. In vitro, this system delivers drug, after an initial short burst, at a controlled rate of 40 to 50 $\mu g/cm^2/hr$ (Figure 9). This value is about one tenth of the initial rate provided by the monolithic dosage form in dissolution testing.

In vitro, the rate of absorption of nitroglycerin from a formulation containing 2% nitroglycerin in ointment, through cadaver skin, is very variable. The rates of nitroglycerin transport can vary (see Table 2) depending upon sex, age, and skin site differences. Thus, placement of a monolithic dosage form puts excess drug in contact with living skin, and the variability in permeation rates observed using cadaver skin is manifest in vivo.

With a multicomponent system, the rate-controlling membrane limits and controls the amount of drug leaving the dosage form and coming in contact with living skin. This control minimizes variations in drug absorption resulting from inherent variations in skin permeability to nitroglycerin. The rate-controlling membrane maintains the drug release rate below the maximum drug permeation rate in living skin, thereby preventing dose-dumping.

Since the advent of this system and other transdermal nitroglycerin dosage forms, the use of the drug to prevent angina has become a routine part of cardiovascular medicine. Patient and physician acceptance of rate-controlled transdermal therapy with Transderm®-Nitro (release rate 5 or 10 mg/day) has been excellent. In one multiweek study of 87 patients, physicians rated the 5 mg/day systems superior to previous therapy (oral nitrates or salves)

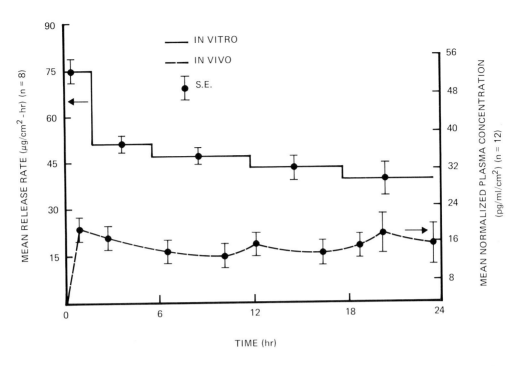

FIGURE 9.   In vitro release rate of nitroglycerin from Transderm®-Nitro on normal skin and plasma concentration resulting from its in vivo application.

Table 2
EFFECTS OF AGE, SKIN SITE, AND SEX ON THE IN VITRO
TRANSEPIDERMAL FLUX OF NITROGLYCERIN (32°C)
PROVIDED BY NITROBID® OINTMENT

Sex	Age (year, ±SD)	Skin Site	Mean flux (μg/hr/cm^2, ±SD)	Range of fluxes (μg/cm^2/hr)	n
Female	72.3 ± 8.6	Hip	10.6 ± 3.2	4.1—16.4	23
	46.6 ± 8.8	Hip	13.4 ± 4.8	8.2—23.0	10
	71.7 ± 6.0	Thigh	7.5 ± 2.5	3.8—10.5	7
Male	71.7 ± 10	Hip	13.5 ± 5.0	9.7—27.0	11
	45.0 ± 12	Hip	13.4 ± 7.3	5.6—25.0	7
	68.9 ± 11	Thigh	13.4 ± 7.3	6.4—27.1	7

in 78% of patients; patient ratings indicated that 66% found transdermal therapy superior.[12]

In a postmarketing surveillance study,[13] the Transderm®-Nitro (5 mg/day) was judged effective in 80.6% of 2461 patients. In addition, the system was well tolerated; 70.5% of the patients had no unwanted effects. The incidences of withdrawals were 5.7% due to headaches, 3.6% from other unwanted effects, and only 3.1% because the treatment was ineffective.

Additional indications may arise in the cardiovascular field for rate-controlled transdermal administration of nitroglycerin. In fact, the ease and precision of the rate-controlled delivery mode makes its use rational for several other drugs in chronic cardiovascular treatment.

VI. TRANSDERMAL CLONIDINE ADMINISTRATION

Hypertension presents several obstacles to faithful compliance with the therapeutic regimen. The disease is usually chronic and predominantly asymptomatic. Oral therapy produces dose-related side effects that can occur several times daily, since hypotensive agents usually require b.i.d. or t.i.d. administration. Noncompliance with such regimens often degrades the use-effectiveness of hypotensive agents relative to their pharmacologic potential.

For clonidine, transdermal therapy represented a rational approach to upgrading use-effectiveness. The drug is potent (oral doses 0.1 to 1.5 mg t.i.d. or b.i.d.), has suitable physicochemical properties for administration through intact skin, and is nonirritating or only mildly irritating to the skin of most patients. Specific therapeutic objectives — in addition to efficacy — were a simplified regimen and side effect reduction to encourage lifelong compliance.

Transdermal clonidine systems provide therapy continuously for 7 days after each application. Drug release rates of 0.1, 0.2, and 0.3 mg/day are available. The rate-controlling membrane used in this system provides a steady-state release of drug, through human skin in vitro, equal to 75% of the rate of drug release into an infinite sink of water.

In patients, one weekly application of the 0.1 mg/day system produces levels of clonidine in plasma that correspond to trough levels of an oral dose of 0.1 mg given twice daily. Compared with oral medication, however, blood concentrations achieved transdermally are more constant (Figures 10 to 12).[14] Steady-state plasma levels of clonidine are reached by the third day after initiation of treatment with both oral and transdermal clonidine. Application of another transdermal system to a fresh skin site immediately after the preceding system is removed maintains steady-state plasma levels continuously. Removal of a system without a replacement causes a gradual decline in blood concentrations of drug.

Among the 69 patients with mild hypertension receiving transdermal clonidine as sole therapy, 48 achieved longterm control of blood pressure. Most patients required use of 0.1 or 0.2 mg/day systems for control of blood pressure. The chief side effects of clonidine therapy — drowsiness and dry mouth — are reportedly reduced by transdermal therapy.[15,16] This may be attributable either to lower daily doses of drug, absence of peaking concentrations of drug in plasma, or both (Figures 10 to 12). Briefly, the advantages obtainable by transdermal clonidine therapy may be summarized as follows:

- Control of hypertension with daily doses lower than those administered orally in many patients
- Seven-day efficacy after each application vs. 12- or 8-hr efficacy with use of tablets
- Side effects reduced in comparison with oral therapy
- Gradual fall in clonidine plasma levels following system removal, preventing rebound hypertension when use is discontinued or when a succeeding dose is delayed

The once-weekly transdermal regimen (vs. 14- or 21-weekly oral doses) and reduced side effects have the potential of increasing patient compliance and thus consistency of longterm hypotensive therapy. In addition, the greater selectivity of action provides the physician with a wider margin for titrating the daily dose up to the optimum hypotensive level. To facilitate these adjustments, the system is available in three strengths programmed to release 0.1, 0.2, or 0.3 mg per day for 1 week.

VII. TRANSDERMAL 17β-ESTRADIOL ADMINISTRATION

A once-daily oral bolus of estradiol has been likened to "hitting the liver with a hammer" every 24 hr,[17] so marked are the elevations in hepatic proteins that result. These elevations have been postulated to cause certain serious side effects of exogenous estrogens, including hypertension, hyperlipidemia, and hypercoagulability.

Oral estrogenic products either are not physiologic hormones or are not administered in

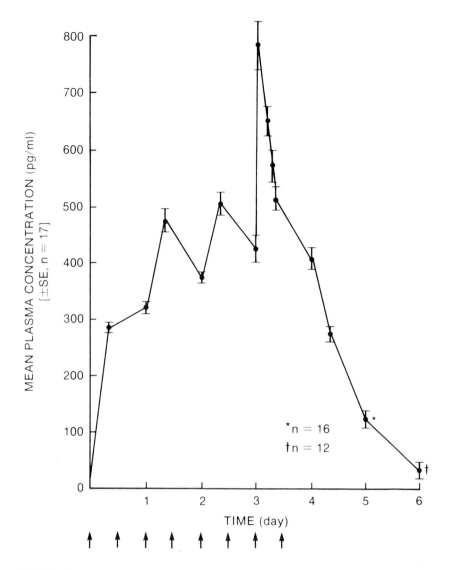

FIGURE 10.   Mean plasma levels of clonidine following administration of oral Catapres® at arrows. Measurements were made twice daily on days 1 to 3 and 5 times on day 4.

a physiologic pattern. Both estradiol (E_2) and conjugated estrogens are substantially metabolized on the first pass through the liver to estrone (E_1) or conjugates. Thus, oral doses must be large to achieve therapeutic estradiol levels and concomitant high levels of circulating E_1 are simultaneously achieved. Moreover, the peak level of the hormone at some point during the dosage interval usually substantially exceeds those prevailing premenopausally.

Estradiol has a plasma half-life of only 1 hour[18] and is not substantially metabolized by skin. Thus, the objectives of rate-controlled transdermal estradiol administration were to present this natural hormone to the body in a pattern mimicking its physiologic secretion — that is, continuously, at a low rate, directly into the bloodstream. Previous parenteral methods — hormone-releasing vaginal rings or creams — appear to raise issues of patient acceptance. In addition, continuous constant-rate transdermal administration offered the prospect of achieving higher E_2 levels and E_2/E_1 ratios from much lower daily doses of E_2 than those given orally.

Rate-controlled (Estraderm™) systems for administering 17β-estradiol through intact skin

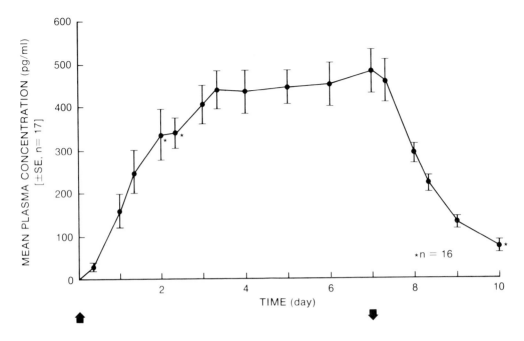

FIGURE 11. Mean plasma concentrations of clonidine during wearing of a 5 cm² Catapres-TTS®. Arrows indicate the time of application and removal of the system.

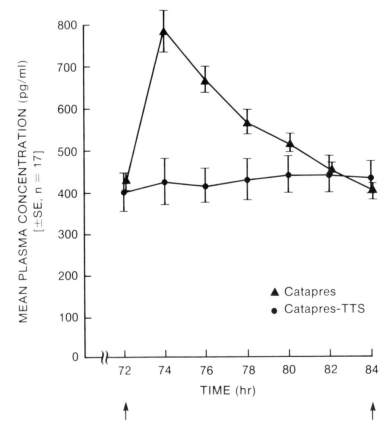

FIGURE 12. Time course of mean plasma concentration of clonidine on day 4 of use of the Catapres-TTS® and oral Catapres®.

Table 3
17β-ESTRADIOL (E_2) AND ESTRONE (E_1) SERUM
CONCENTRATION INCREMENTS AND E_2/E_1 RATIOS
AFTER 3 DAYS OF E_2 ADMINISTRATION

Route and dose of estradiol	Mean increase above baseline (pg/mℓ)		Ratio E_2/E_1
	17β-Estradiol	Estrone	
Oral			
2 mg/day	59	303	0.19—0.25
Transdermal			
0.025 mg/day	16	0.3	
0.05 mg/day	32	9	0.9—1.4
0.1 mg/day	67	27	

are applied twice weekly. They are programmed to release, in vivo, 0.025, 0.05, or 0.1 mg estradiol per day, according to patients' needs.

A study in postmenopausal women[19] — with pretreatment E_2 and E_1 levels in serum of 7.4 pg/mℓ and 32.3 pg/mℓ, respectively — showed that following system application therapeutic E_2 levels in serum were achieved in less than 4 hr and persisted during the entire system wearing. The E_2/E_1 ratio was elevated and maintained in the premenopausal range. Within 24 hr after removal of the systems, serum concentrations of E_2 and E_1 returned to untreated levels. In contrast, orally administered 17β-estradiol (2 mg/day) produced mean peak levels of E_2 and E_1 of 133 pg/mℓ and 709 pg/mℓ, respectively, 8 hr after administration. Table 3 shows the rises in serum concentrations of E_2 and E_1 resulting from administration by the two different routes.

In a placebo-controlled 3-week study, menopausal women experiencing frequent hot flashes (measured by digital thermography) used transdermal systems delivering 0.05 mg or 0.10 mg estradiol per day;[20,21] systems were replaced twice weekly. In patients who received the larger systems, measurements were also made of vaginal cytology, plasma gonadotropins, hepatic proteins, and urinary calcium/creatinine ratios.

In patients receiving the 0.05 mg and 0.10 mg systems, circulating E_2 levels rose respectively fivefold (to an average of 38 pg/mℓ) and tenfold (average of 72 pg/mℓ). These E_2 plasma concentrations are equivalent to those observed during the early follicular phase in premenopausal women. Hot flashes decreased from 0.79/hr and 0.76/hr to 0.35/hr and 0.25/hr, respectively. E_2/E_1 ratios in both groups increased to those typical of the premenopausal range.

Transdermally administered estradiol exerted positive effects on vaginal cytology; the percentage of superficial cells was significantly increased. Follicle-stimulating hormone and luteinizing hormone levels decreased significantly. Blood pressure was not affected during this 3-week period.

No significant increases in the concentration of renin substrate or other hepatic proteins (sex hormone-binding globulin, thyroxine-binding globulin, and corticosteroid-binding globulin) occurred. Thus, transdermal estradiol does not effect the changes in the hepatic function known to occur with oral administration of conjugated and synthetic estrogens.

In summary, rate-controlled transdermal estradiol administration appears to offer several advantages over the oral route:

- Maintenance of controlled, therapeutically effective, physiologic levels of E_2 with low daily doses of 17β-estradiol
- Maintenance of physiologic E_2/E_1 ratios
- Rapid clearance of E_2 and its metabolites after removal of systems, providing a ready pause in estrogen therapy when cycling is desirable
- A convenient twice-weekly regimen vs. daily bolus dosing

VIII. CONCLUSION

A new family of transdermal dosage forms has been developed that provides rate-controlled administration of drugs to the systemic circulation. Transdermal systems have been developed that deliver scopolamine, nitroglycerin, clonidine, and 17β-estradiol. Each of these dosage forms was designed to fulfill specific therapeutic needs and to optimize the pharmacologic properties of the drug.

The systems described here improve treatment by simplifying regimens and maintaining steadier plasma levels of drug than is possible with oral dosage forms. Because these dosage forms are the products of new technology, they required the development of methods of manufacture new to the pharmaceutical industry.

REFERENCES

1. **Shaw, J. and Urquhart, J.,** Programmed, systemic drug delivery by the transdermal route, *Trends Pharmacol. Sci.*, 1, 208, 1980.
2. **Shaw, J. E. and Urquhart, J.,** Transdermal drug administration — a nuisance becomes an opportunity, *Br. Med. J.*, 283, 875, 1981.
3. **Shaw, J. E.,** Transdermal dosage forms, in *Drug and Enzyme Targeting Part A*, Methods of Enzymology, Vol. 112, Widder, K. J. and Green, R., Eds., Harcourt, Brace & Jovanovich, Orlando, Fla., 1985, 448.
4. **Shaw, J. E. and Dohner, J. W.,** Transdermal dosage forms from ALZA, *Manuf. Chem.*, 53, 1985.
5. **Weiner, N.,** Atropine, scopolamine, and related antimuscarinic drugs, in *Goodman and Gilman's The Pharmacological Basis of Therapeutics*, 6th ed., Gilman, A. G., Goodman, L. S., and Gilman, A., Eds., MacMillan, New York, 1980, 120.
6. **Money, K. E.,** Motion sickness, *Physiol. Rev.*, 50, 1, 1970.
7. **Brand, J. J. and Perry, W. L. M.,** Drugs used in motion sickness, *Pharmacol. Rev.*, 18, 895, 1966.
8. **Price, N. M., Schmitt, L. G., McGuire, J., Shaw, J. E., and Trobough, G.,** Transdermal scopolamine in the prevention of motion sickness at sea, *Clin. Pharmacol. Ther.*, 29, 414, 1981.
9. **Schmitt, L. G., Shaw, J. E., McGuire, J., and Thorn, D.,** Effect of drugs on vertigo induced by caloric irrigation of the external auditory canal, *Clin. Pharmacol. Ther.*, 29, 282, 1981.
10. **Babin, R. W., Balkany, T. J., and Fee, W. E.,** Transdermal scopolamine in the treatment of acute vertigo, *Ann. Otol. Rhinol. Laryngol.*, 93, 25, 1984.
11. **Shaw, J. E.,** Development of the transdermal therapeutic system, presented at a seminar on Transdermal Therapeutic System: A Major Advance in Angina Prophylaxis, in conjunction with the 16th Annu. American Soc. Hospital Pharmacists Midyear Clinical Meeting, New Orleans, December 6, 1981.
12. **Garnier, B., Imhof, P., Spinelli, F., and Jost, H.,** Field study: treatment of angina pectoris with a new transdermal therapeutic system containing nitroglycerin, under practice conditions, *Schweiz. Rundsch. Med.*, 71, 511, 1982.
13. **Bridgman, K. M., Carr, M., and Tattersall, A. B.,** Post-marketing surveillance of the Transiderm-Nitro patch in general practice, *J. Int. Med. Res.*, 12, 40, 1984.
14. **Arndts, D. and Arndts, K.,** Pharmacokinetics and pharmacodynamics of transdermally administered clonidine, *Eur. J. Clin. Pharmacol.*, 26, 79, 1984.
15. **Popli, S., Stroka, G., Ing, T. S., Daugirdas, J. T., Norusis, M. J., Hano, J. E., and Gandhi, V. C.,** Transdermal clonidine for hypertensive patients, *Clin. Ther.*, 5, 624, 1983.
16. **McMahon, F. G., Michael, R., Jain, A., and Ryan, J. R.,** Clinical experience with clonidine TTS, in *Mild Hypertension: Current Controversies and New Approaches*, Weber, M. A. and Mathias, C. J., Eds., Steinkopff Verlag, Darmstadt, W. Germany, 148, 1984.
17. **Campbell, S. and Whitehead, M. I.,** *The Controversial Climacteric*, MTP Press, Lancaster, England, 103, 1981.
18. **Nichols, K. C., Schenkel, L., and Benson, H.,** 17β-Estradiol for postmenopausal estrogen replacement therapy, *Obstet. Gynecol. Surv.*, 39, 230, 1984.
19. **Powers, M. S., Schenkel, L., Darley, P. E., Good, W. R., and Balestra, J. C., and Place, V. A.,** Pharmacokinetics and pharmacodynamics of transdermal dosage forms of 17β-estradiol: comparison with conventional estrogen used orally for hormone replacement, *Am. J. Obstet. Gynecol.*, 152(8), 1099, 1985.
20. **Laufer, L. R., DeFazio, J. L., Lu, J. K. H., Meldrum, D. R., Eggena, P., Sambhi, M. P., Hershman, J. M., and Judd, H. L.,** Estrogen replacement therapy by transdermal estradiol administration, *Am. J. Obstet. Gynecol.*, 146, 533, 1983.
21. **Steingold, K. A., Laufer, L., Chetkowski, R. J., DeFazio, J. D., Matt, D. W., Meldrum, D. R., Judd, H. L.,** Treatment of hot flashes with transdermal estradiol administration, *J. Clin. Endocrin. Metab.*, 61, 627, 1985.

Chapter 9

TRANSDERMAL DELIVERY OF NITROGLYCERIN FROM A POLYMERIC GEL SYSTEM

G. Cleary and A. Keith

TABLE OF CONTENTS

I. INTRODUCTION

Patients have been using nitroglycerin (NTG) to relieve the pain inflicted by angina pectoris since 1879 when William Murrell established its use in acute anginal episodes and as well as its prophylactic ability in preventing recurring pain.[1] For quick relief, absorption of NTG through the mucous membrane beneath the tongue has been the most popular mode of administration. However, because of the severity of the anginal pain and the short half-life of NTG, a patient would have to take several tablets at once and quite frequently and the blood levels would be quite high and erratic. Attempts of controlling the blood level by oral ingestion have been unsuccessful because of NTG's rapid metabolism in the liver ("first-pass" effect). In the 1950s, NTG in the form of an ointment was tried clinically and soon found a place in angina therapy that allowed for a sustained coverage of about 6 hr.[2] Problems encountered with the ointment have been the inconvenience (greasiness and several steps necessary to apply to the skin) and irreproducibility of the amount applied by the patient. More recently an intravenous (i.v.) dosage form has reached the market. Although the i.v. product can only be used in nonambulatory patients in the hospital, it does allow for a continuous blood level by intravenous drip. As can be seen, NTG therapy has exhibited a need for improved delivery to the patient over the years.

The transdermal approach provided by the ointment was in the right direction but was not ideal. NTG provides an example of a drug that is an ideal candidate for a transdermal system. NTG has a very short half-life of 1 to 3 min and up to 60% is degraded in the liver after oral ingestion.[3] The liver is the first metabolic unit that NTG sees after absorption through the gastrointestinal wall. Drugs permeating through skin do not go directly to the liver and have an opportunity to survive longer, thus making them able to exert greater specific activity. The amount of NTG needed to exert a pharmacological effect is small. It takes less than 500 μg to treat angina sublingually.

Prior to the development of Nitro-Dur®, the permeation rate of NTG through skin, in vitro, has been reported in the literature to be in a range from 10 to 25 mcg/cm^2/hr at steady state.[4] These skin flux data were obtained using saturated solutions of NTG.

In vivo studies in man have been reported in the literature whereby 2% ointment was spread over areas ranging from 25 to 100 cm^2. Maier-Lenz, et al. achieved peak blood levels with 30.4 mg NTG (1% ointment) in 30 min with a blood level of 0.53 ng/mℓ.[5] Blood levels were not detectable at 2 hr. Armstrong et al.,[6] reported higher blood levels of about 3 ng/mℓ with a 2% ointment over 58 cm^2. Sved and his co-workers also studied the ointment dosage form and considered the effect of area of application and total amount applied.[7] They essentially found peak blood levels of 0.17 and 0.41 ng/mℓ for volunteers receiving 25 and 10 cm^2 of 2% NTG ointment (16 mg total). A single application of the ointment lasted for about 6 hr. To achieve high enough blood levels one would have to assume that the patient would have to reapply the ointment every 4 to 5 hr each day.

Since it is well established that NTG permeates the skin and is useful in treating anginal pain by that route, it would be a useful task to improve the delivery of NTG such that the patient could be treated with fewer applications per day, eliminate the vagaries of the ointment dosage form and simplify the number of steps needed to apply the NTG to the skin. Key Pharmaceuticals, Inc., has developed a 25-hr transdermal system for nitroglycerin (Nitro-Dur®) as shown in Figure 1.

In the development of Nitro-Dur®, it is useful to understand the diffusional characteristics of NTG both in its polymeric matrix as well as through the skin. In the design of the system, one not only considers the permeation parameters of NTG, but also the adhesional properties of the components, the packaging aspects, the functional properties of the skin, and most importantly, the pharmacokinetics and pharmacodynamics of NTG in the body.

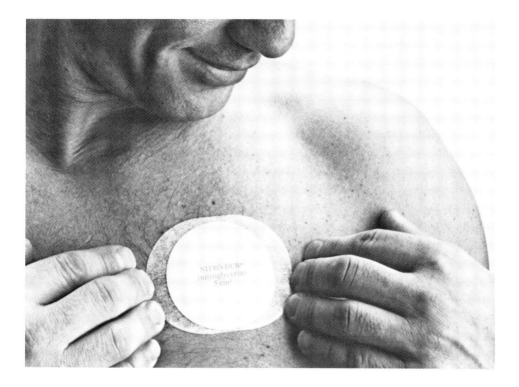

FIGURE 1.   Nitro-Dur® transdermal infusion system being applied to the skin (courtesy of Key Pharmaceuticals, Inc.).

II. IN VITRO STUDIES

Diffusion is usually thought of as taking place over a concentration gradient; however, diffusion is a general phenomenon which describes the translational motion of atoms, molecules, or particles. The diffusing species must be small enough to be susceptible to Brownian motion. The extent of diffusion (rate) of a given species is well described by the Debye equation for rotational motion given by

$$\tau_c = \frac{4\pi r^3 \eta}{3kT} \tag{1}$$

and the Stokes-Einstein equation for diffusion,

$$D = \frac{kT}{6\pi r \eta} \tag{2}$$

where τ_c is rotational correlation time, η is viscosity (poise), k is Boltzman constant, T, temperature in °K, r, radius of, or spherical equivalent of species in centimeters, and D, diffusion (cm²/sec).

Both these equations describe molecular motion resulting from kT/η and are further limited by properties of the diffusing species.

Application of these equations to heterogeneous environments is not straightforward because barriers to diffusion may exist which limit diffusion over macrodimensions more than over microdimensions.

Experiments to describe the diffusional properties existing in the Key Pharmaceutical Nitro-Dur® diffusion matrix were investigated using three separate methods of determining the diffusion coefficient of small molecules.

Two molecules were used which have some structural homology and the same general size as NTG. The two molecules shown below have been extensively investigated in biochemical, biophysical, and chemical physical experiments.

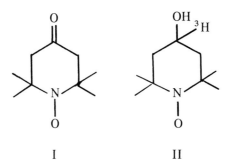

I   II

Both these spin label probe molecules result in three electron spin resonance (ESR) absorption lines when the condition for resonance is satisfied. This condition is described by:

$$h\nu = g\beta H, \tag{3}$$

where h is Boltzman constant, ν is the applied microwave frequency, β is the Bohr Magneton, H is the applied magnetic field intensity usually expressed in gauss, and g is a constant determined by ν and H. Under proper conditions, both these probe molecules give rise to three resonance absorption lines. The nature of the local environment is reflected in the relative heights and widths of these three absorption lines. Information relative to local viscosity, physical binding, local polarity, collisional frequency of probe molecules, rotational motion, and translational motion can be obtained in well-defined experiments.

For present purposes, the rotational correlation time (τ_c) of I is measured in Nitro-Dur® and collision frequency between probe molecules is derived from measurements of the probe collision frequency of I at higher concentrations.

The rotational correlation time (τ_c) of I was determined in the Nitro-Dur® diffusion matrix at 24°C by application of

$$\tau_c = 6.5 \times 10^{-11} \, W_o \left[\left(\frac{h_o}{h_{-1}} \right)^{1/2} - 1 \right] \tag{4}$$

where W_o is mid field line width, h_o is mid field line height, and h_{-1} is high field line height.

The τ_c measured was 0.5×10^{-10} sec using a probe concentration of 1 mM and reflects an environment of relatively low viscosity, about three times that of water.

Combining Equations 1 and 2 allows for a diffusion coefficient (D) to be calculated in terms of rotational motion (D_τ).

$$D_\tau = \frac{0.67 \, r^2}{\tau_c} \tag{5}$$

The value of D_τ is limited by the rotational motion of I. If the forces that limit molecular motion are the same over very small dimensions (in the neighborhood of 5 to 10 Å) as they are over considerably larger dimensions (50 to 500 Å) then D_τ will be a realtively accurate measurement of a diffusion coefficient (D).

The calculated value for D_τ is 2.2×10^{-6} cm²/sec.

The same probe was also used at considerably higher concentrations, 40, 50, and 60 mm. At these concentrations in Nitro-Dur® at 24°C collision frequency between probe molecules is adequately high to broaden all three resonance lines. The concentration dependent line broadening is a measure of collision frequency by the well-studied mechanism known as electron spin exchange (ω_{ex}). The relation relating diffusion of the probe molecule to spin exchange frequency (ω_{ex}) has been well established where

$$D_c = k \frac{\omega_{ex}}{[M]} \tag{6}$$

ω_{ex} is electron spin exchange frequency often expressed by concentration line dependent broadening, (ΔH). ω_x can be converted to frequency unit by multiplying ΔH by a conversion number, 2.8×10^6 cycles/sec/gauss. Thus, ω_{ex} is expressed in terms of cycles/sec. Then, D_c can be solved with a simplified form of Equation 6 expressed as

$$D_c = 5.6 \times 10^{-8} \frac{\Delta H}{[M]} \tag{7}$$

where D_c is the diffusion coefficient arrived at by measuring collision frequency and where the constant 5.6×10^{-8} is arrived at by experiments carried out on tritiated probe II.[8] In these experiments, the diffusion constant of probe II was determined in water under conventional conditions[8] and then Equation 6 was solved for the constant ($k = 5.6 \times 10^{-8}$). ΔH is the peak-to-peak measured line width minus the line width in the same environment at very low probe concentrations.

The value of D_c arrived at for Nitro-Dur® after application of this treatment is $D_c = 9.7 \times 10^{-7}$ cm²/sec.

A third method was used for measuring diffusion of a water soluble dye in Nitro-Dur® (FD&C Blue #1). One preparation of Nitro-Dur® was made containing 1% dye; another preparation was made containing no dye. Segments of both were cut with a razor and one dyed segment was placed in diffusional contact with an undyed segment. The preparation was incubated in a petri plate at 24°C and diffusion boundary measurements were made at intervals for 24 hr. The data were plotted as dye diffusion distance (s) against the square root of time $(t)^{1/2}$ in seconds. The collected data allowed application of the equation

$$s^2 = 2Dt \tag{8}$$

to solve for D. For this case, the measured diffusion coefficient will be called bulk diffusion (D_b). This diffusion value was calculated to be 5.5×10^{-7} cm²/sec.

Comparison of these three measured or derived diffusion values illustrates interesting properties of heterogeneous environments. These three values,

$$D_b = 5.5 \times 10^{-7} \text{ cm}^2/\text{sec}$$

$$D_c = 9.7 \times 10^{-7} \text{ cm}^2/\text{sec}$$

$$D_\tau = 2.2 \times 10^{-6} \text{ cm}^2/\text{sec}$$

all illustrate important features of molecular motion and diffusional properties. All three of these methods of measurement agree in general when carried out on the same or similar solvents. The reason for agreement is that water and other fairly isotropic solvents have a relatively homogenous environment. A polymer gel, however, is a heterogenous preparation having a polymer lattice with solvent zones comprised of small molecules filling the space not occupied by polymers. The polymers present barriers to diffusion and the higher percentage of the polymer the more of an obstacle the polymer molecules present to diffusing species. If the polymers are so crowded together that small molecules cannot pass between polymers except occasionally the diffusion is greatly reduced. Rotational motion, however, may not be so impeded as translational motion; therefore D_r derived from τ_c measurements gives the impression of a more fluid environment than bulk phase diffusion measurements.

Molecular motion in heterogeneous polymer preparations sometimes results in surprising findings. For example, a preparation where polymers in solvent solution on suspension are induced to phase separate and form local laminates or precipitates then the final preparation is formed of two phases. The solvent phase and the polymer phase are now separated in space. Over molecular dimensions, diffusion occurs rapidly within solvent zones and much more slowly between solvent zones that are separated by polymer aggregates or layers.

Such a system was investigated using Bio Rad® column chromatography polyacrylamide beads designated as P2, P6, P30, and P100. The P notation designates the limiting pore size for macromolecular flow through the bead structure. For example, P2 excludes all macromolecules of approximately greater than 2,000 daltons and P100 excludes molecules of greater than 100,000 daltons. These beads, therefore, apparently form a gradient of pore sizes. At a density of one these beads have a limiting spherical equivalent pore size of a diameter of

$$P2, 19 \text{ Å},$$
$$P6, 27 \text{ Å},$$
$$P30, 47 \text{ Å},$$
$$\text{and,} \quad P100, 68 \text{ Å}.$$

Using probe I and P2 beads the diffusion coefficient calculated by using probe collision frequency (D_c) at four concentrations are the following:

Molarity	Probe cubic lattice spacing (Å)	D (cm²/sec)
0.030	55	2×10^{-7}
0.044	34	2×10^{-7}
0.067	29	3×10^{-7}
0.100	26	5×10^{-7}

This clearly points out that for a matrix having fixed pore dimensions with limiting size channels or pores that collision frequency between probe molecules is probe concentration dependent. As the probe concentration increases, the probability of having more than one probe per "cavity" increases. Again this points out that molecular motion may be relatively rapid in local fluid zones but that translational diffusion between fluid zones may be dramatically impeded by polymer barriers.

These general considerations are particularly important when taking high percentage polymer matrices such as adhesives into account. Most adhesives are composed of highly anisotropic polymers. This film spreading of these adhesives solubilized or dispersed in a volatile solvent may result in an anisotropic film where more polymer molecules have the long axis of symmetry parallel to the thin film than perpendicular to the thin film. This anisotrophy may be important when a transdermal device is covered with or is primarily composed of adhesive. The implication of this consideration is that two diffusion coefficients exist, that is, a diffusional coefficient, $D_\parallel$, parallel to the plane of the adhesive, and a diffusion coefficient perpendicular to the plane of the adhesive, $D_\perp$.

III. SYSTEM DESIGN

In the development of the Nitro-Dur® transdermal infusion system, one can essentially divide the critical parts into four separate areas:

1. Aluminum foil package
2. Polymer/nitroglycerin matrix
3. Adhesional components
4. Absorbance pad

A. Aluminum Foil Package

In the case of Nitro-Dur®, the package is part of the system. The matrix contains NTG and other liquids that potentially could evaporate from the matrix. These volatile components should be surrounded by packaging materials which will not allow them to escape during the lifetime of the system on the shelf. A well-known barrier, aluminum foil, completely surrounds the matrix material as shown in Figure 2A with a baseplate and a removable coverstrip. The heat seal is designed with appropriate peel characteristics such that the coverstrip can be removed exposing the matrix (Figure 2B). The foil baseplate remains behind on the system to serve as a barrier to NTG and the other liquid components while the patient is wearing the system. The foil is flexible enough to be worn and machinable during manufacture.

B. Polymer/Nitroglycerin Matrix

The polymer matrix serves as the substrate that contains the nitroglycerin until it is ready to be released. The formulation of the matrix must be designed so that the NTG is available to the skin for permeation through the stratum corneum. One can consider both the diffusional characteristics of NTG in the matrix and the skin on the micro- or macrolevel. The polymeric matrix of Nitro-Dur® is composed of polyvinyl alcohol (PVA) and polyvinyl pyrrolidone (PVP) to form the lattice structure with the interstitial spaces filled with a mixture of liquid components. The microdiffusional parameters have been discussed earlier and elsewhere where the rotational and translational diffusional coefficients are described for the fluid phase and the polymeric structure.[9] From this information one can determine the effect of increasing or decreasing the cross-linking of the two polymers, PVA and PVP, on the release of the NTG. A permeation rate of 40 to 45 μg/cm^2 NTG was observed from the Nitro-Dur® matrix into the placebo matrix (same formulation except that it contains no NTG).[9] The macrodiffusional characteristics indicate that the skin permeability of NTG from the matrix remains constant for over 48 hr at about 20 μg/cm^2/hr (Figure 3). This flux value is similar to those found in the literature where NTG was applied to the skin in saturated solutions and other transdermal systems.[4,10] The amount of NTG in the Nitro-Dur® matrix is sufficient to maintain a saturated solution in the fluid phase for the required 24 hr. As shown in Equation 9, the flux will remain constant as long as C_m remains constant and $D_m \gg D_s$

$$\text{Flux} = J_s = \frac{K_{s/m} \, D_s \, C_m}{\delta} \tag{9}$$

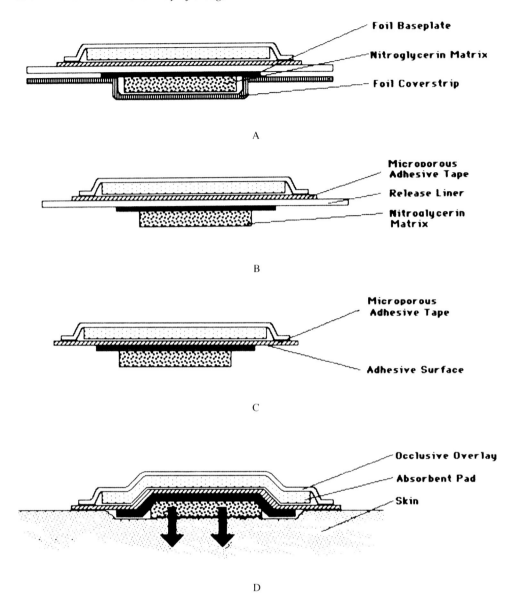

FIGURE 2.   System design of Nitro-Dur® (schematic diagram). (A) Nitro-Dur® self-contained package unit; (B) foil coverstrap removed, exposing NTG matrix; (C) release liner removed, exposing adhesive surface; system is ready to apply to the skin; (D) Nitro-Dur® system placed on the skin.

where $K_{s/m} = C_s/C_m$ = partition coefficient of NTG dissolved in the skin and NTG dissolved in the matrix.

C_s = concentration of NTG in the skin
C_m = concentration of NTG in the matrix
δ = thickness of limiting layer of skin
D_s = diffusion coefficient of NTG in the skin, cm²/sec
D_m = diffusion coefficient of NTG in the matrix, cm²/sec

By adjusting the formula of the matrix one can change, in principle, the values of the permeation parameters to obtain the desired flux within limits.

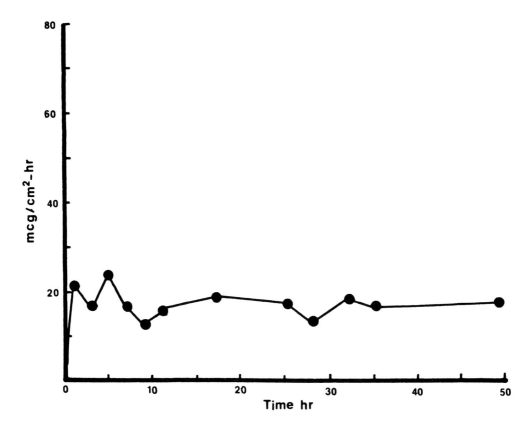

FIGURE 3.   In vitro flux of NTG through human cadaver skin at 37°C, n = 3.[8]

C. Adhesional Components

There are several adhesional aspects of the various components used in Nitro-Dur® that are important to the function of the system while it is being readied for application and while it is being worn on the skin. Once the coverstrip is removed, the release liner must be removed (Figure 2B) to expose the pressure sensitive adhesive that holds the Nitro-Dur® system to the skin (Figure 2C). The formulation of the adhesive and the release liner has to be optimized to allow for ease of opening and fabrication of system (Figure 4). While the adhesive on the tape layer must allow for easy release from the protective release liner, it must adhere to the baseplate with great tenacity when the coverstrip is removed but not so great as to damage the skin when it is removed from the skin (Figure 2A and D). Once the system is applied to the skin, the adhesive must remain on the skin for 24 hr. During this interim, the tape is confronted with water, perspiration, oils, and the contours and stretching motion of the skin. The pressure sensitive adhesive must be all things to several layers at the same time. Finally, the occlusive overlay (Figure 2D) must adhere to the backside of the adhesive tape during the 24-hr wearing interval and while the absorbent pad is collecting fluid.

The selection of proper adhesive for the Nitro-Dur® involved consideration of the adhesive-cohesive properties, peel strength, tack, and creep qualities of candidate adhesives. The stability of the adhesive strength and other properties is as important as the stability of NTG in the development of the system. Adhesion definitions as they apply to transdermals have been reviewed elsewhere.[11]

D. Absorbent Pad

There can be a build-up of perspiration, particularly in hot weather, beneath the Nitro-

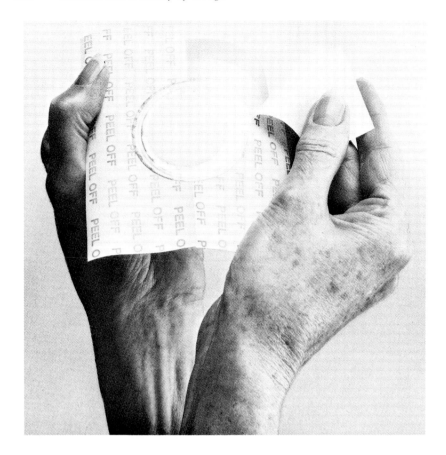

FIGURE 4.   Release liner being removed from the Nitro-Dur® Transdermal Infusion System (courtesy of Key Pharmaceuticals, Inc.).

Dur® system during the wearing interval. A nonocclusive adhesive tape has been incorporated into the Nitro-Dur® system to allow movement of any excess fluid from the site of application (Figure 2C). A certain amount of fluid at the matrix/skin interface helps to maintain a bridge between the matrix and the skin, thus allowing for permeation of NTG through the skin. However, an absorbent pad has been placed on one side of the porous tape to soak up the excess fluid. The fluid reaches the absorbent pad by permeating around the baseplate, through the porous tape and into the absorbent pad. The occulsive overlay prevents further migration of the excess fluid. The periphery of the Nitro-Dur® adhesive is nonocclusive as well to allow perspiration to be vented. This helps in maintaining good adhesion of the system while the patient is wearing Nitro-Dur®.

IV. CLINICAL EVALUATIONS

A. Pharmacokinetics

Nitro-Dur® has been tested on human volunteers to study blood levels and its pharmacological effects. Mazoyer and Darbeau showed that in 18 healthy male volunteers, a constant blood level was achieved between 30 min and 32 hr.[12] The plateau levels reached were 236 ± 32 pg/mℓ with a 20 cm² system. Golub et al. similarly found a mean plasma concentration of 200 pg/mℓ with a 20 cm² system (Figure 5).[12] Similar blood levels have been found with other transdermals (on a per cm² basis).[10] The blood levels remain constant over the 24-hr period in all transdermals whether there is a claim of membrane control or not. Similar zero-

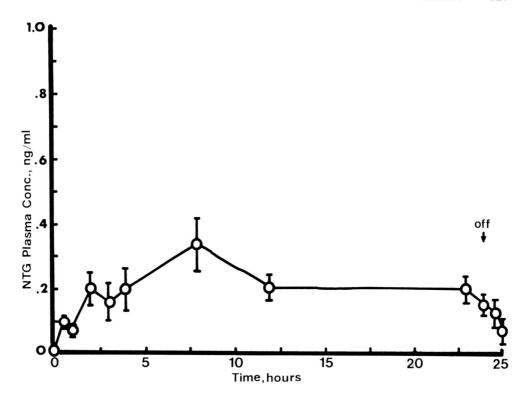

FIGURE 5.   Mean NTG plasma concentration time profile in six normal volunteers.[12]

Table 1
NITRO-DUR® DOSAGE SIZES

NTG matrix surface area, (cm²)	NTG content, (mg)	NTG delivered over 24 hr (mg)
5	26	2.5
10	51	5.0
15	77	7.5
20	104	10.0

order (constant) kinetic profiles have been obtained in vitro with Nitro-Dur® as well as the other membrane controlled transdermals.[4,10] Based on the values of skin flux in the literature from saturated solutions of NTG and similar blood levels achieved by other commercially available transdermals (even those claiming membrane controlled release), it appears that the skin is the rate controlling element in all cases. Table 1 lists the different sizes of Nitro-Dur® currently available on the market along with the NTG content and the amount delivered in 24 hr. As can be seen from Table 1, there is excess NTG available compared to the amount delivered in 24 hr. This excess NTG will accommodate any loss of NTG through any excess perspiration or to effect a change in the thermodynamic driving force, e.g., maintaining a unit activity equal to one.

B. Pharmacodynamics

Along with the information gathered with the pharmacokinetic data, a series of ongoing studies are being performed to study the efficacy of the transdermal nitroglycerin in the treatment of angina pectoris. One clinical method of determining efficacy is accomplished by exercise testing. Here, the patient develops a work level by exercising on a treadmill or bicycle and the onset of anginal pain is recorded with and without administration of nitroglycerin. In a study of six men with stable angina pectoris, no anginal episodes occurred after 4, 10, and 28 hr after Nitro-Dur® application when the work load increased in the range of 32 to 37%.[14] In another study, Pucci et al., found that Nitro-Dur® (20 cm², 104 mg) enabled 10 subjects to increase their workload on a bicycle exerciser of greater than 44% than without the drug.[15] In the same study, a long-acting isosorbide dinitrate preparation (20 mg every 8 hr) increased the workload by greater than 37%. Nitro-Dur® maintained its beneficial action consistantly for 21 hr. Schiavoni and others performed a similar study with Nitro-Dur® (20 cm², 104 mg) in 12 subjects suffering with angina pectoris.[16] They found that the quantity of work performed increased by 41% at the 6th hr ($p < 0.0001$) compared to controls and by 39% at the 24th hr ($p < 0.0001$). The average total duration of exercise before the onset of anginal pain was 360 ± 80 sec in the control but increased to 510 ± 78 sec and 500 ± 69 sec at the 6th and 24th hr, respectively with Nitro-Dur®. In a treadmill study, Hollenberg and Go found that Nitro-Dur® (5, 10, 15, and 20 cm²) improved the treadmill exercise score (derived from an index that quantifies the ST-segment response to exercise) by 31% ($p < 0.0001$).[17] The dose response on the treadmill exerciser for the different sizes of Nitro-Dur® was very weak as has been demonstrated with other nitrate preparations. Other potential indications have been reported with Nitro-Dur®, such as its use in the treatment of congestive heart failure.[18]

V. SUMMARY

In the body of this treatment, we have dealt with the events that lead to the transdermal use of NTG and the criteria for efficacious transdermals using NTG. Some of the important considerations are release rate from matrix, skin permeability, patient acceptance, and overall quality of patient therapy.

The general structural features of an NTG transdermal delivery system are important and improvements are expected to be made until physical and physiological limits are reached. These considerations are total size, reliability, efficacy, and dose control. Adhesives are, in principle, ideal for the delivery of transdermals because adhesives allow close contact between delivery surface and skin surface. Adhesives are frequently composed of high percentage polymers which dramatically impede diffusion processes. Adhesives need a substantial fluid phase to allow adequate diffusion of dry and an appropriate three-dimensional lattice to allow passage of drug without limiting barriers. Adhesives also need modification so as to allow solubility control over the drug of interest.

The Nitro-Dur® transdermal system was initially constructed without adhesive contact between the delivery surface and skin because available adhesive systems impeded diffusion of NTG and reduced the small flux.

REFERENCES

1. **Murrel, W.,** Nitroglycerin as a remedy for angina pectoris, *Lancet,* 1, 80, 1879.
2. **Davis, J. A. and Wissel, B. G.,** *Am. J. Med. Sci.,* 230, 259, 1955.
3. **Needleman, P., et al.,** The metabolism pathway in the degredation of glycerol trinitrate, *J. Pharmacol. Exp. Ther.,* 179, 347, 1971.
4. **Micheals, A. S., Chandrasekaran, A. K., and Shaw, J. E.,** Drug permeation through human skin: theory in vitro experimental measurement, *A.I.Ch.E. J.,* 21, 985, 1975.
5. **Maier-Lenz, V. H., Ringwelski, L., and Windorfer, A.,** Pharmacokinetics and relative bioavailability of a nitroglycerin ointment formulation, *Arzneim. Forsch.,* 30, 320, 1980.

6. **Armstrong, P. W., Armstrong, J. A., and Marks, G. S.,** Blood levels after sublingual nitroglycerin, *Circulation,* 59, 585, 1979.
7. **Sved, S., McLean, W. M., and McGilveray, I. J.,** Influence of the method of application on pharmokinetics of nitroglycerin from ointment in humans, *J. Pharm. Sci.,* 70, 1368, 1981.
8. **Keith, A. D., Snipes, W., Melhorn, R. J., and Gunter, T.,** Factors restricting diffusion of water-soluble spin labels, *Biophys. J.,* 19, 205, 1977.
9. **Keith, A. D.,** Polymer matrix considerations for transdermal devices, *Drug Dev. Ind. Pharm.,* 9, 605, 1983.
10. **Black, C. D.,** Transdermal drug delivery systems, *U.S. Pharm.,* 7, 49, 1982.
11. **Cleary, G. W.,** Transdermal controlled release systems, in *Medical Applications of Controlled Release,* Langer, R. and Wise, D., Ed., CRC Press, Boca Raton, Fla., 1984, 203.
12. **Mazoyer, F. and Darbeau, D.,** A study of the bioavailability of glycerol trinitrate administered transcutaneously to healthy volunteers using a specific assay, presented at a Symp. Preceding the American College of Cardiology Annual Meeting, New Orleans, March 19, 1983.
13. **Golub, A. L., Gonzalez, M. A., and Blanford, M. F.,** Evaluation of the absorbtion kinetics of nitroglycerin following application of the Nitro-Dur® system, presented at a Symp. Preceding the American College of Cardiology Annual Meeting, New Orleans, March 19, 1983.
14. **Sellier, P., Audouin, P., Payen, B., Corona, P., and Maurice, P.,** Therapeutic efficacy of a new transcutaneously absorbed nitroglycerin in stable angina pectoris, evaluated by exercise testing, presented at a Symp. Preceding the American College of Cardiology Annual Meeting, New Orleans, March 19, 1983.
15. **Pucci, P., Zambaldi, G., Cerisano, G., and Roccanti, P.,** Evaluation of a new preparation of transdermal nitroglycerin for patients with angina of effort, *G. Ital. Cardiol.,* 13, 167, 1983.
16. **Schiavoni, G., Mazzari, M., Lanza, G., Frustaci, A., Mongiardo, R., and Pennestri, F.,** Evaluation of the efficacy and the length of action of a new preparation of slow-release nitroglycerin for percutaneous absorbtion (Nitro-Dur®, Sigma Tau) in angina pectoris caused by exercise, *Int. J. Clin. Pharm. Res.,* 2(2), 15, 1982.
17. **Hollenberg, M. and Go, M.,** Efficacy of transdermal nitroglycerin patches in patients with angina pectoris, *Cardiovas. Rev. Rep.,* 9, 1984.
18. **Olivari, M. T., Carlyle, P. F., Levine, T. B., and Cohn, J. N.,** Hemodynamic and humoral response to transdermal nitroglycerin in congestive heart failure, *Clin. Res.,* 30, 548, 1982.

Chapter 10

TRANSDERMAL ABSORPTION OF NITROGLYCERIN VIA A MICROSEALED DRUG DELIVERY SYSTEM

Aziz Karim

TABLE OF CONTENTS

I. INTRODUCTION

Nitroglycerin (NTG) is a potent, lipophilic, neutral drug with a low molecular weight. It undergoes extensive first-pass metabolism following oral administration[1] and it has a short elimination half-life of about 3 min, a high apparent distribution volume of about 3 ℓ/kg, and a high plasma clearance of about 0.7 ℓ/min.[2] These physicochemical and pharmacokinetic properties make NTG an ideal candidate for administration by the transdermal route. A topical dosage form of NTG is already available as a 2% ointment.[3,4] The ointment, however, is messy to use and the applied dose, based on the concentration and the surface area, may vary[5,6] markedly from day to day.

II. FORMULATION ASPECTS OF MDD-NTG (Nitrodisc®) SYSTEM

The controlled-release NTG transdermal systems currently marketed fall into two main categories: those in which the drug is stored in a membrane sealed reservoir and those in which the drug is stored in a matrix. The "Microseal Drug Delivery" (MDD) system, developed by G. D. Searle & Co., combines the principles of the reservoir and matrix systems.

Details of formulation and manufacturing of the MDD-NTG system appear in the U.S. Patent.[7] The MDD-NTG system (Figure 1) contains a silicone polymer matrix affixed to an aluminum backing. The silicone polymer matrix has cross-linked silicone rubber with numerous microsealed compartments. These microcompartments are formed *in situ* as a result of cross-linking of the liquid silicone rubber polymer during emulsification between the hydrophilic solvent system (polyethylene glycol 400 in distilled water containing the NTG) and the hydrophobic solvent system, e.g., isopropyl palmitate. The hydrophobic system enhances NTG transport and dispersion through the silicone polymer matrix allowing diffusion of NTG at a constant rate when the MDD-NTG system is placed on the skin.

The matrix is composed of silicone polymers represented by the formula

$$\left[\begin{array}{c} CH_3 \\ | \\ O{-}Si{-} \\ | \\ CH_3 \end{array}\right]_n \quad \begin{array}{c} R \\ | \\ {-}O{-}Si{-}O{-} \\ | \end{array} \left[\begin{array}{c} CH_3 \\ | \\ Si{-}O \\ | \\ CH_3 \end{array}\right]_n$$

$$\left[\begin{array}{c} O \\ | \\ CH_3{-}Si{-}O{-} \\ | \\ CH_3 \end{array}\right]_n$$

wherein R is alkoxy, alkyl, phenyl, vinyl, or allyl and n is about 100 to 5000.

In preparing the MDD-NTG system, a uniform paste is made of a NTG-lactose mixture, polyethylene glycol 400, and distilled water. This paste is then added to the silicone elastomer along with the appropriate amount of a hydrophobic solvent. These ingredients are mixed in a low shear, explosion-proof mixing vessel maintained under a vacuum. The polymerizing catalyst is added and mixing is continued under vacuum. The viscous mixture thus formed is poured into clean, dry stainless steel plates, and placed in an air circulating oven at about 60°C. After 2 hr of curing, the MDD-NTG pad adhering to the aluminum foil is pulled off, cut into suitable size pads, e.g., 2 × 4 cm with aluminum foil backing. The pads are then stored in air tight containers as described in the U.S. Patent. The above description is for laboratory-scale preparation of the MDD-NTG system. The currently marketed Nitrodisc® is manufactured by a fully automated process.

A

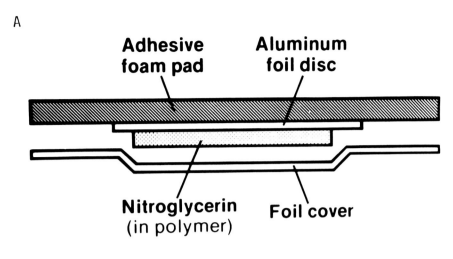

Adhesive foam pad   **Aluminum foil disc**

Nitroglycerin (in polymer)   **Foil cover**

B

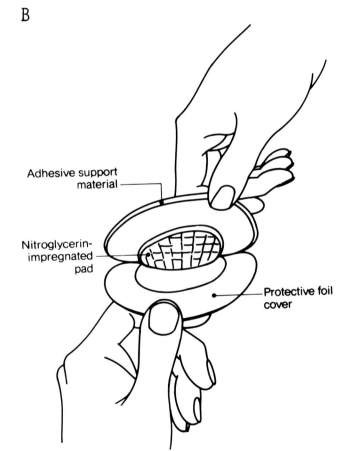

Adhesive support material

Nitroglycerin-impregnated pad

Protective foil cover

FIGURE 1. Microseal Drug Delivery-Nitroglycerin (MDD-NTG; Nitrodisc®). (A) Cross-section of MDD-NTG system, (B) circular MDD-NTG system. The 8 cm^2 system contains 16 mg NTG (2 mg/cm^2) and the 16-cm^2 system contains 32 mg NTG (2 mg/cm^2), (C) electron micrograph of MDD-NTG system illustrating the presence of microcompartments which serve as tiny reservoirs for nitroglycerin.

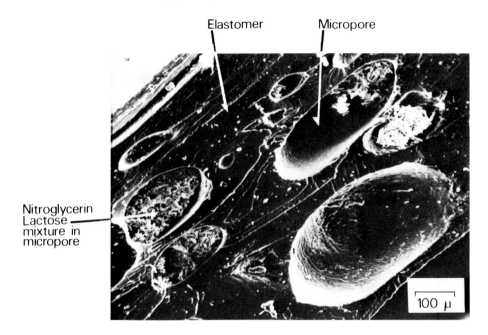

FIGURE 1C

III. BIOPHARMACEUTICAL ASSESSMENT OF MDD-NTG (Nitrodisc®) SYSTEM

There are several practical problems in evaluating transdermal absorption of NTG such as:

- The reference standard of NTG is not available as a pure crystalline material but as a 10% NTG lactose adsorbate. The standard curve for the assay should therefore be prepared with pure substance collected by sublimation and weighed.
- NTG is rapidly adsorbed to[8] and hydrolyzed by[9] red blood cells. Therefore, immediate inhibition of the hydrolases, centrifugation, and extraction of plasma samples following blood collection is necessary.
- The therapeutic plasma levels of NTG are very low (<1 ng/mℓ) so a highly accurate and sensitive assay method capable of detecting 0.05 ng/mℓ level is required.
- NTG has numerous side effects including headache, postural hypotension, flushing, tachycardia, and dizziness. The dose of NTG used in a human bioavailability study therefore cannot be too high; otherwise the subject dropout rate may be excessive.

In the studies described below, plasma levels of NTG were determined by a quantitative gas-liquid chromatographic method using isosorbide dinitrate as the internal standard and electron capture detection.

A. NTG Release Rate When in Contact with Human Skin

The currently marketed MDD system for nitroglycerin (MDD-NTG; Nitrodisc®) contains 16 mg NTG over 8 cm^2 and 32 mg NTG over 16 cm^2. The kinetics of NTG release in vivo in healthy subjects to whom the MDD-NTG patch (16 mg NTG over 8 cm^2) was applied on the chest is shown in Figure 2. In six subjects, a mean $\pm$ SD of 1.22 $\pm$ 0.71, 1.60 $\pm$ 1.19, 3.42 $\pm$ 1.01, and 4.99 $\pm$ 1.16 mg of NTG was released over 3, 6, 12, and 24 hr, respectively. These findings indicate that the in vivo release of NTG from the MDD-NTG system occurs in a slow and controlled manner.

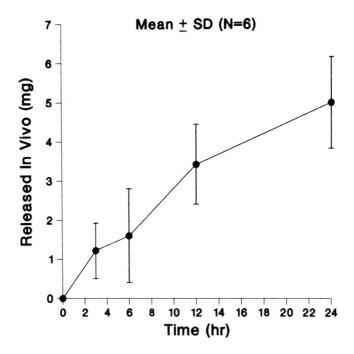

FIGURE 2.   In vivo release of nitroglycerin at various time periods in six healthy subjects following application of MDD-NTG (16 mg NTG over 8 cm²) on the chest.

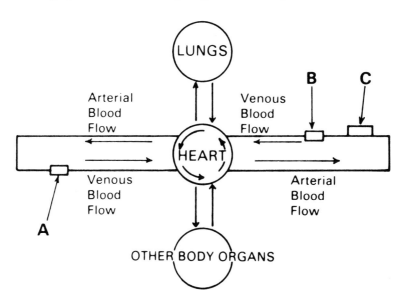

FIGURE 3.   Procedure for evaluating transdermal absorption of nitroglycerin in man. MDD-NTG is applied on the volar surface of the wrist (C) and NTG plasma levels are determined in the ipsilateral (B) and the contralateral (A) forearm antecubital veins.

B. NTG Absorption Rate In Vivo

A simple and useful method of studying transdermal absorption of drugs is outlined in Figure 3. A test preparation of known surface area and concentration per square centimeter is applied on the volar surface of the wrist and the time course of plasma drug concentrations is determined simultaneously in the antecubital vein of the forearm bearing the test preparation (ipsilateral) as well as the opposite arm (contralateral). High ipsilateral plasma levels represent

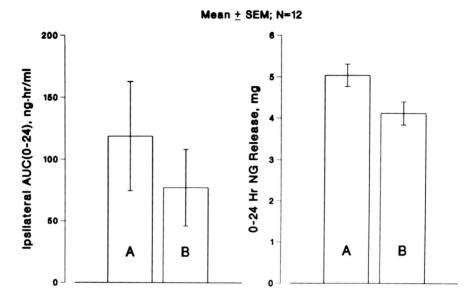

FIGURE 4.   Relationship between mean 0 to 24 hr ipsilateral AUC (ng.hr/mℓ) and mean 24-hr NTG release (mg) following application of Nitrodisc® or MDD-NTG on the volar surface of the wrist. (A) Nitrodisc® (16 mg NTG over 8 cm²), (B) MDD-NTG (16 mg NTG over 8 cm²).

drug concentration near the site of absorption while the low contralateral plasma levels represent systemic concentrations. This method, therefore, permits evaluation of the time course of the systemic plasma concentrations as well as the plasma concentrations near the site of absorption.

Using the above technique we have evaluated the basic transdermal absorption characteristics of NTG. Clinical studies were performed in a randomized, crossover manner in healthy male subjects. Test preparations constituted 4 to 16 cm² of MDD-NTG systems containing 4 to 32 mg of NTG and 1/2 to 2 in. of 2% NTG ointment (Nitro-Bid®, Marion Laboratories, Inc., Kansas City, Mo.) spread over approximately 53 cm². The major findings from these studies are summarized below.

1. Amount of NTG Released vs. Amount Absorbed

Figure 4 illustrates the relationship between the amount of NTG released from two formulations of MDD-NTG, each containing 16 mg NTG over 8 cm², and the amount absorbed through the skin of 12 healthy male subjects. The amount of NTG absorbed through the skin, as represented by the area under the ipsilateral plasma concentration-time curve (AUC), was related to the amount of NTG released from MDD-NTG. Release measurements when in contact with skin, therefore, provide a quick and reliable method of checking bioavailability of NTG from different MDD-NTG formulations. Furthermore, the variability in the measurement of amount released was considerably lower than the variability in AUC measurement. Therefore, small differences in the bioavailability of a test formulation can be more reliably detected by the former method.

2. Surface Area and Transdermal Absorption

Figure 5 illustrates the ipsilateral plasma levels of NTG as the surface area of the applied MDD-NTG containing 2 mg NTG per cm² is increased from 4 to 16 cm². An approximately linear relationship was found between the ipsilateral AUC and the surface area of the applied MDD-NTG.

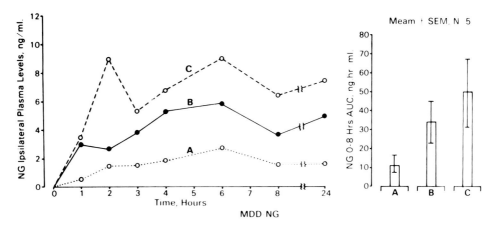

FIGURE 5. Relationship between the surface area of the application site and the ipsilateral plasma levels of nitroglycerin. Each value is a mean of five healthy male subjects and vertical bars represent SEM. MDD-NTG systems were applied on the volar surface of the left wrist in a crossover study. (A) 8 mg NTG over 4 cm^2 (2 mg/cm^2), (B) 16 mg NTG over 8 cm^2 (2 mg/cm^2), (C) 32 mg NTG over 16 cm^2 (2 mg/cm^2).

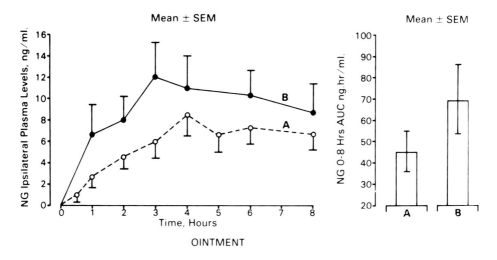

FIGURE 6. Relationship between the concentration and the ipsilateral plasma levels of nitroglycerin. 2% Nitro-Bid® ointment was applied over a fixed area on the volar surface of the left wrist. (A) 1/2 in, 8 mg NTG over 53 cm^2 (0.15 mg/cm^2), N = 23, (B) 1 in, 16 mg NTG over 53 cm^2 (0.30 mg/cm^2), N = 6.

3. Concentration and Transdermal Absorption

With a constant surface area of about 53 cm^2, ipsilateral plasma levels increased by approximately 1.5 times when the concentration of NTG applied on the skin as an ointment was increased from 0.15 to 0.30 mg/cm^2 (Figure 6). It must be emphasized, however, that this finding applies only to the concentration range studied: saturation in transdermal absorption is very likely at higher concentrations of NTG (2 mg/cm^2) as present in the MDD-NTG system.

4. Factors to be Considered in Computing Bioavailability

Figure 7 represents hypothetical curves illustrating the influence of changing either the surface area of the application site or the dosage strength (mg/cm^2) of the transdermal preparation on the plasma concentration of NTG. Assessment of this relationship is necessary in choosing an optimally bioavailable transdermal dosage form of a test drug. Also, both the concentration and surface area difference should be considered when comparing bioavailability of the test drug from different transdermal preparations.

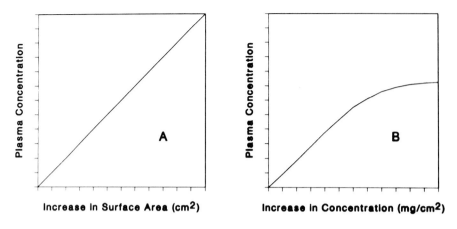

FIGURE 7.   Hypothetical pattern illustrating relationship between the surface area of the application site and the drug concentration on the transdermal absorption. (A), the concentration (mg/cm²) is kept constant; (B), the surface area (cm²) is kept constant.

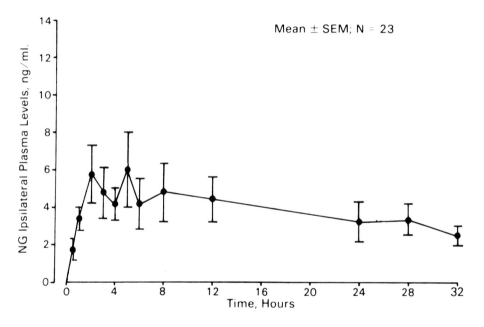

FIGURE 8.   Ipsilateral plasma concentration-time curve of nitroglycerin in healthy male subjects following application of MDD-NTG (16 mg over 8 cm²) on the volar surface of the left wrist.

5. Intersubject Variability in Transdermal Absorption

Figure 8 demonstrates the mean ± SEM ipsilateral plasma levels of NTG over a period beyond 24 hr in 23 subjects in whom MDD-NTG (16 mg over 8 cm²) was placed on the volar surface of the wrist. Slow and continuous absorption of NTG occurred resulting in about 4 ng/mℓ constant mean ipsilateral plasma levels for a period of up to 32 hr. A high between-subject variability was found in the transdermal absorption of NTG and this variability was attributed largely to the differences in the skin characteristics of individuals since there was a statistically significant correlation between the ipsilateral AUC with MDD-NTG and the ointment (Figure 9).

6. Is There Retention of NTG to the Skin?

Figure 10 illustrates decrease in ipsilateral plasma concentrations 1 hr after removal of

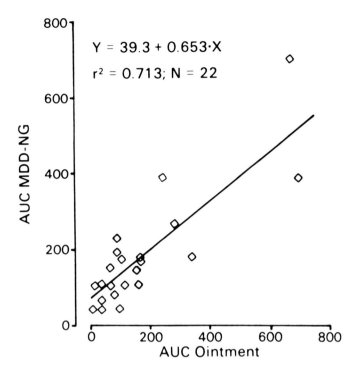

FIGURE 9.   Relationship between 0 to 48 hr ipsilateral area under the plasma concentration-time curves (AUC, ng/hr/mℓ) with MDD-NTG (16 mg over 8 cm^2) and
2% ointment (8 mg over 53 cm^2) applied on the volar surface of the left wrist.

MDD-NTG pads. Ipsilateral plasma levels decreased by 66% (from 1.79 $\pm$ .39 to 0.60 $\pm$
.13 ng/mℓ) 1 hr after removing the pad. Significant retention of NTG to the skin is therefore
not present.

7. Systemic Plasma Levels

In the study design outlined in Figure 3, systemic plasma levels of NTG in the contralateral
arm were found to be below the detection limit of the assay following application of the
highest dose of either MDD-NTG (32 mg NTG over 8 cm^2) or ointment (1 in. [16 mg] over
53 cm^2). The transdermal absorption of NTG was therefore re-examined using the same
doses of MDD-NTG and Nitro-Bid ointment applied on the precordial region of the chest
in a randomized, balanced, crossover study in 12 healthy subjects.

With the chest application, systemic NTG plasma levels of about 0.3 ng/mℓ in the left
and the right forearm veins were similar and were maintained for a period of 24 hr and
beyond (Figure 11). These findings suggest that a site-related difference exists in the systemic
availability of the transdermally applied NTG and that for optimal pharmacological response,
topical NTG preparations should not be applied on the distal part of the body. A similar
conclusion was also made by Hansen et al.[10] who noted significant pharmacological differences in the responses of normal subjects to NTG ointment when the same dose was applied
to different body sites.

8. Relationship Between In Vivo Release of NTG from Matrix and Reservoir Transdermal Systems

The importance of an individual's skin rather than the release mechanism of NTG in the
transdermal absorption of NTG was highlighted in a randomized crossover study in which
two patches of Transderm®-Nitro 5 (each patch = 25 mg NTG over 10 cm^2) or two patches

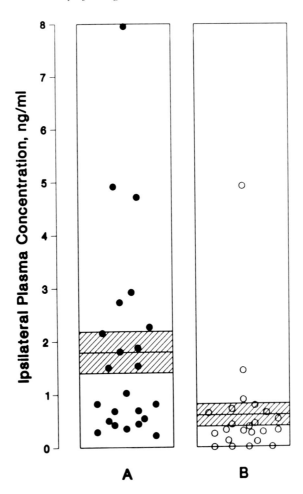

FIGURE 10.   Ipsilateral plasma concentrations of NTG in 23 subjects at 48 hr (A) and 1 hr after removal (B) of MDD-NTG patch containing 16 mg NTG over 8 cm². The MDD-NTG patch was applied on the volar surface of the wrist for 48 hr. Horizontal lines represent mean values and shaded areas ± SEM.

of Nitrodisc® (each patch = 16 mg NTG over 8 cm²) were applied for 24 hr on the chests of 16 adult healthy male subjects. The mean ± SD in vivo release of NTG from each Nitrodisc® and Transderm®-Nitro 5 was 5.4 ± 2.0 mg and 6.2 ± 1.7 mg (P > 0.05), respectively (Figure 12). Furthermore, a weak but statistically significant correlation was found between the total amount of NTG released in vivo from two patches of Nitrodisc® (matrix system) and two patches of Transderm®-Nitro 5 (reservoir system) (Figure 13). This correlation suggests that it was the skin and not the device release mechanism that was the rate-determining factor in how much NTG was available for absorption in vivo.

IV. LABELING FOR TRANSDERMAL SYSTEMS

The introduction of transdermal NTG patches by three different companies [Nitrodisc® (Searle), Transderm®-Nitro (Ciba/Geigy), and Nitro-Dur® (Key)] makes it desirable to have uniform product labeling (Table 1). The most important information that a physician needs to know is how much NTG is delivered to the patient over the 24-hr dosing interval. Table 1 shows that even though the NTG content and surface area of the currently marketed transdermal products differ widely, the average amounts of NTG released in vivo in 24 hr

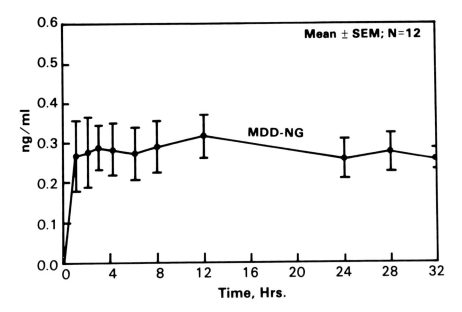

FIGURE 11.   Mean systemic plasma concentration-time curve of nitroglycerin in 12 healthy male subjects following application of MDD-NTG (32 mg over 16 cm^2) on the precordial region of the chest.

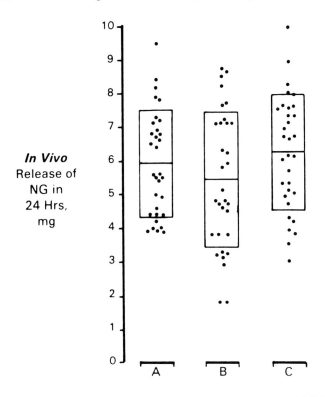

FIGURE 12.   Release of nitroglycerin in vivo (mean ± SD; N = 32) with MDD-NTG, Nitrodisc®, or Transderm®-Nitro 5. Two patches of each preparation were applied on the chest of 16 healthy subjects for 24 hr in a randomized, crossover study. (A) MDD-NTG; 16 mg NTG over 8 cm^2, (B) Nitrodisc; 16 mg NTG over 8 cm^2, (C) Transderm-Nitro 5; 25 mg NTG over 10 cm^2.

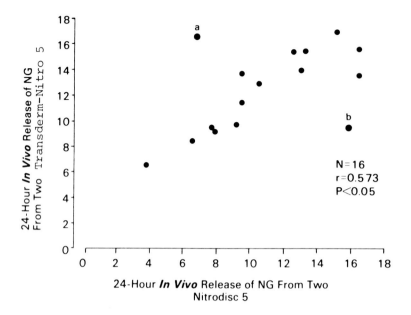

FIGURE 13.   Relationship between the total amount of NTG released in vivo in 24 hr from two patches of Nitrodisc® 5 (each patch = 16 mg NTG over 8 cm²) and two patches of Transderm®-Nitro 5 (each patch = 25 mg NTG over 10 cm²) applied on the chests of 16 healthy male subjects. The r value of 0.901 was obtained when data for two outliers a and b were excluded from the regression analysis.

Table 1
COMPARISON OF TRANSDERMAL NITROGLYCERIN (NTG) PRODUCTS

Product name	Manufacturer	Product surface area (cm²)	NTG content (mg)	Average amount of NTG delivered in vivo (mg/24 hr)
Transderm®-Nitro 5	Ciba	10	25	5.0
Transderm®-Nitro 10	Ciba	20	50	10.0
Nitro-Dur® 5	Key	5	26	2.5
Nitro-Dur® 10	Key	10	51	5.0
Nitro-Dur® 15	Key	15	77	7.5
Nitro-Dur® 20	Key	20	104	10.0
Nitrodisc® 5	Searle	8	16	5.0
Nitrodisc® 10	Searle	16	32	10.0

are similar. It should be stressed, however, that the in vivo release rate values given in Table 1 are approximate average values and, as pointed out before, an individual's skin is the rate-limiting factor in determining the amount of NTG available systemically.

REFERENCES

1. **Armstrong, P. W., Armstrong, J. A., and Marks, G. S.,** Blood levels after sublingual nitroglycerin, *Circulation,* 59, 585, 1979.
2. **McNiff, E. F., Yacobi, A., Young-Chang, F. M., Golden, L. H., Goldfarb, A., and Fung, H.-L.,** Nitroglycerin pharmacokinetics after intravenous infusion in normal subjects, *J. Pharm. Sci.,* 70, 1054, 1981.

3. **Franciosa, J. A., Blank, R. C., Cohn, J. N., and Mikulic, E.,** Hemodynamic effects of topical, oral, and sublingual nitroglycerin in left ventricular failure, *Curr. Ther. Res., Clin. Exp.,* 22, 231, 1977.

4. **Armstrong, P. W., Armstrong, J. A., Marks, G. S., McKinven, J., and Slaughter, S.,** Pharmacokinetic-hemodynamic studies of nitroglycerin ointment in congestive heart failure, *Am. J. Cardiol.,* 46, 670, 1980.

5. **Sved, S., McLean, W. M., and McGilveray, I. J.,** Influence of the method of application on pharmacokinetics of nitroglycerin from ointment in humans, *J. Pharm. Sci.,* 70, 1368, 1981.

6. **Kirby, J. A. and Woods, S. L.,** A study of variation in measurement of doses of nitroglycerin ointment, *Heart Lung,* 10, 814, 1981.

7. **Sanvordeker, D. R., Cooney, J. G., and Wester, R. C.,** U.S. patent 4,336,243, 1982.

8. **Wu, C., Sokoloski, T., Blanford, M. F., and Burkman, A. M.,** Absence of metabolite in the disappearance of nitroglycerin following incubation with red blood cells, *Int. J. Pharm.,* 8, 323, 1981.

9. **Armstrong, J. A., Slaughter, S. E., Marks, G. S., and Armstrong, P. W.,** Rapid disappearance of nitroglycerin following incubation with human blood, *Can. J. Physiol. Pharmacol.,* 58, 459, 1980.

10. **Hansen, M. S., Woods, S. L., and Wills, R. E.,** Relative effectiveness of nitroglycerin ointment according to site of application, *Heart Lung,* 8, 716, 1979.

Chapter 11

TRANSDERMAL DELIVERY FROM SOLID MULTILAYERED POLYMERIC RESERVOIR SYSTEMS

Agis F. Kydonieus

TABLE OF CONTENTS

ABSTRACT

Transdermal delivery systems are new polymeric devices for administering medication through the skin. The Hercon Division, through its agreements with a dozen major pharmaceutical companies, is working toward the transdermal delivery of several pharmaceutical agents, using a patented[1] system, composed of at least three solid polymeric layers.

I. THE DEVICE

A schematic cross-section of a typical Hercon laminated membrane structure is shown in Figure 1. One of the outer layers is completely impervious to the active ingredient while the other outer layer is the one that contacts the skin and controls the release of the active ingredient from the system. A pressure sensitive adhesive is attached to the impervious or barrier layer to secure the system onto the skin. The specially formulated inner layer, which behaves as the reservoir, contains dissolved drug which then migrates continually due to imbalance of chemical potential through the initially inert outer layer to the surface rendering it biologically active. When in contact with human skin, the drug dissolves in the skin tissue and diffuses into the body.

The construction and composition of the laminated membranes vary, of course, with the drug used, release rate, and effective life span desired. However, materials containing from 0.5% to 40%, by weight, drug have been successfully prepared and have been shown to be efficacious in a number of in vitro as well as in vivo experiments.

The Hercon laminated reservoir system is uniquely suited for use in transdermal applications because:

1. It is a very flexible system and can control the release by using different polymers in the reservoir and protective layers
2. It can give zero-order release for the useful life of the system
3. It can accommodate solid or liquid drugs
4. It eliminates the possibility of dose "dumping"
5. It can be manufactured inexpensively and rapidly
6. It can be fabricated to be extremely thin and, therefore, produce acceptable bioavailabilities for drugs with very low doses

II. THE MATHEMATICS OF TRANSPORT

The class of membranes used with the Hercon technology is the nonporous, homogeneous polymeric films. These membranes are usually referred to as solution-diffusion membranes. Silicone rubber, polyethylene, polyvinyl chloride, and nylon films are typical examples.

The drug is able to pass through the membrane material in the absence of pores or holes by a process of absorption, solution, diffusion down a gradient of thermodynamic activity, and desorption. The process of permeation is thus divisible into a number of independent processes governed primarily by Fick's law.[2,3]

$$J = -D \frac{d C_m}{dx} \tag{1}$$

where J is the flux in $g/cm^2/sec$, C_m is the concentration of drug in the membrane in g/cm^3, dC^m/dx is the gradient in concentration, and D is the diffusion coefficient of the drug in the membrane in cm^2/sec.

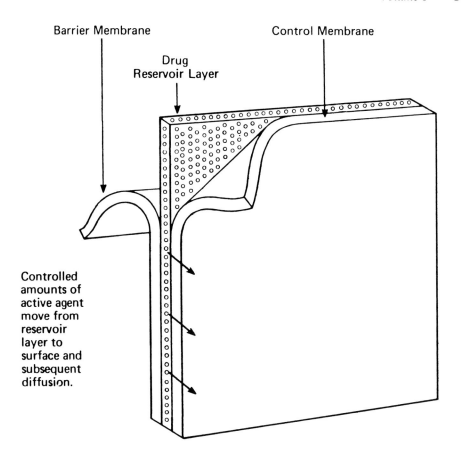

FIGURE 1.   The Hercon controlled release transdermal dispenser.

A. The Zero-Order Device

As shown in Figure 2, the concentration just inside the membrane surface can be related to the concentration in the reservoir C by the expressions:

$$C_{m(0)} = KC_{(0)} \text{ at the upstream surface } (x = 0)$$

$$C_{m(1)} = KC_{(1)} \text{ at the downstream surface } (x = 1) \tag{2}$$

where, K is a distribution coefficient and is analogous to the familiar liquid-liquid partition coefficient. In Figure 2, for purposes of illustration, it has been assumed that the distribution coefficient is less than unity for control membrane I, and more than unity for control membrane II. Throughout the following, we will assume diffusion coefficients and distribution coefficients to be constant. This is a safe assumption for most polymer-drug systems. Thus, in the steady state, Equation 1 can be integrated to give

$$J = D \frac{Cm_{(0)} - Cm_{(1)}}{1} = D \frac{\Delta C_m}{1} \tag{3}$$

where 1 is the thickness of the membrane. Since the concentration within the membrane is usually not known, Equation 3 is frequently written:

$$J = \frac{dM_t}{Adt} = \frac{DK \, \Delta C}{1} \tag{4}$$

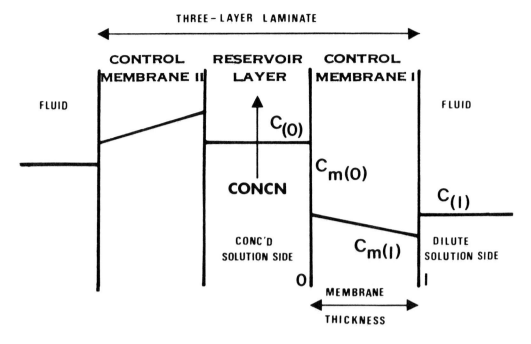

FIGURE 2.   Schematic representation of the concentration gradient across a three-layer laminate.

where M_t is the mass of agent released, dM_t/dt is the steady state release rate at time t and ΔC is the difference in concentration ($C_{(0)}$ to $C_{(1)}$) between the reservoir concentration and the fluid concentration adjacent to the control membrane. It is significant to note that the rate of release is proportional to the diffusivity (a kinetic constant) and to the distribution coefficient (a thermodynamic constant). Equation 4 can be integrated between the limits:

$$M_t = 0 \quad t = 0$$

$$M_t = M_t \quad t = t$$

$$\text{to give } M_t \quad = \frac{ADK\ \Delta C}{l} t \tag{5}$$

When the distribution coefficient between the reservoir layer and the control membrane is much smaller than unity, as is the case of membrane I in Figure 2, the system has excellent release kinetics and the release rate can be maintained constant for extended periods of time (pseudo-zero order delivery). Equation 5 is then governing the process and a straight line is obtained when the mass of agent released (M_t) is plotted against time (t).

B. The Half-Order Device

When the distribution coefficient between the reservoir layer and the control membrane is approximately unity, or larger than unity, as is the case with membrane II of Figure 2, the system will approximate the "dissolved system", i.e., the reservoir-control membrane system forms a single homogenous polymeric film. The concentration in the reservoir will not remain constant but will fall continuously with time. The system remains continuously under unsteady-state conditions and the mass of agent released varies as a function of time (half order of delivery). The transport equations have been described by several investigators.[4,5]

The two useful equations are the early time approximation, which holds over the initial portion of the curve,

$$\frac{M_t}{M_\infty} = 4\left(\frac{Dt}{\Pi l^2}\right)^{1/2} \quad 0 \leqslant \frac{M_t}{M_\infty} < 0.6 \tag{6}$$

and the late time approximation, which holds over the final portion of the release curve,

$$\frac{M_t}{M_\infty} = 1 - \frac{8}{\Pi^2} \exp\left(\frac{-\Pi^2 Dt}{l^2}\right) \quad 0.4 \leqslant \frac{M_t}{M_\infty} \leqslant 1.0 \tag{7}$$

As it can be seen from Equation 6, a plot of the mass of agent released vs. time will give a parabolic curve.

III. FACTORS AFFECTING THE RELEASE

Looking at Equations 5, 6, and 7, it becomes apparent that the release of active ingredients from Hercon laminated membrane structures is controlled by molecular and structural factors.[6] For a given combination of polymer structure and active agent where energy of free rotations, free volume, and intermolecular attractions are constant, at least two parameters are available to regulate the rate of transfer, reservoir concentration and membrane thickness.

Diffusivity D and reservoir/membrane distribution coefficient K are also directly proportional to the permeation rate. In polymers, diffusivity is strongly sensitive to the molecular weight of the diffusant and to the stiffness of the backbone of the polymeric membrane. Simply speaking, the diffusant molecule will have to reorient several segments of polymer chain to allow its passage from site to site. The higher the molecular weight, the more the segments that need to be reoriented for passage to be possible; and the stiffer the polymer (glassy and high crystallinity), the more difficult for its segments to undergo large reorientations. Therefore, variables that could affect the stiffness of polymer membranes such as codiffusants that would soften, plasticize, or partially dissolve the membrane would have an effect on diffusivity and permeation rate.

The reservoir/membrane distribution coefficient K can be estimated from the solubility parameter of the diffusant. Solubility parameters can be calculated using Hilderbrand's solubility theory. When the solubility parameters for the diffusant and polymer membrane are the same, the polymer will be soluble in the diffusant. The solubility parameters and dissolution are strongly affected by molecular weight and the chemical functionality of the molecule, i.e., hydrogen bonding and polarity.

In Figures 3 and 4 the effect of reservoir concentration and control membrane thickness on the permeation of the skin enhancer Deet is shown. The dramatic effect of molecular weight on permeation is illustrated in Figure 5 for a homologous series of acetates. Finally the distribution of the fungicide Captan between a flexible polyvinyl chloride film and polymer films of increasing backbone stiffness is shown in Table 1.

IV. DEVELOPMENT OF A NITROGLYCERIN PATCH — INITIAL STUDIES

A. Dissolution Studies

Three separate experiments were performed. In the first experiment, the effect of nitroglycerin concentration in the patch on its dissolution under infinite sink conditions was investigated. As expected, the amount of nitroglycerin released was higher at the higher concentrations of nitroglycerin in the patch (Table 2).

In the second experiment, the effect of polymer modifiers on the dissolution rate was

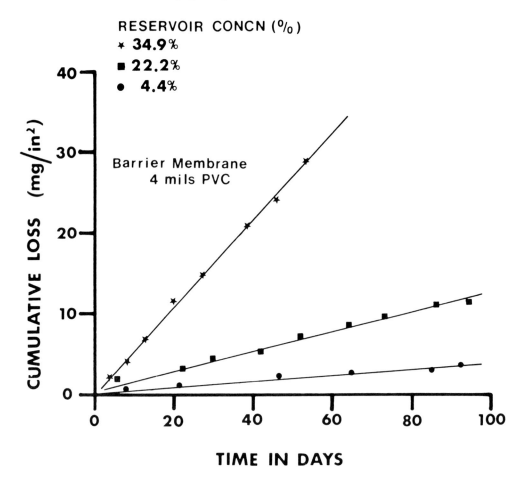

FIGURE 3.   Effect of reservoir concentration on release of deet.

studied. Table 3 indicated that modifiers can have a significant effect on the release of nitroglycerin.

In the third experiment, a representative Hercon patch was tested side by side with the three commercial nitroglycerin patches. The results shown in Table 4 indicate that more nitroglycerin is released from the Hercon patch than from the Ciba and G. D. Searle patches, but lower than from the Key patch.

In all of the above experiments, the dissolution studies were performed under infinite sink conditions, in Hanson dissolution equipment with a rotational speed of 100 rpm at 37°C. The nitroglycerin content was obtained by determining the amount of nitroglycerin in the sink fluid by the Bratton-Marshall technique. The base polymers used in the manufacture of all patches were PVC copolymers and terpolymers.

B. In Vitro Skin Penetration

The penetration of nitroglycerin from the Hercon patch was measured through cadaver skin at 31°C. In Figure 6, the average cumulative penetration of nitroglycerin flux is 15 ± 7 $\mu g/cm^2$/hour, which agrees with values in the literature.

These experiments were performed with isolated human female abdominal epidermis, and 20% polyethylene glycol 400 in water was used as the receptor phase to maintain sink conditions. Nitroglycerin was quantitated by HPLC using a PRP-1 column (Hamilton) and acetonitrile:water (55:45) as the mobile phase.

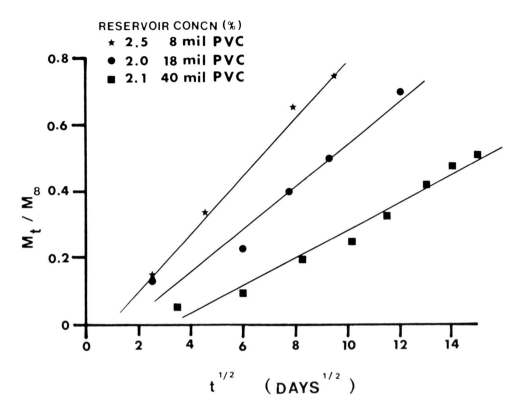

FIGURE 4.   Effect of control membrane thickness on release of deet.

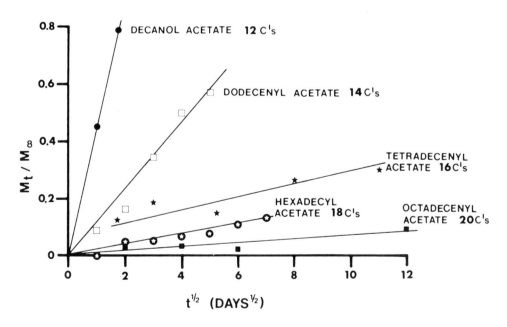

FIGURE 5.   Effect of molecular weight on mass of agent released.

Table 1
DISTRIBUTION OF ACTIVE AGENT BETWEEN FLEXIBLE PVC AND POLYMERS OF INCREASING BACKBONE STIFFNESS

	Active agent transported (ppm)				
	Flex PVC[1]	Rigid PVC	Polyprop	Nylon	Polyester
Captan	50	109	36	3	0

[1] All polymer films were 5-mil thick. The total amount of captan in the system was 500 ppm. Readings were taken 20 weeks after the initiation of experiment.

Table 2
EFFECT OF NTG CONCENTRATION ON DISSOLUTION

% NTG	2.00	5.00	10.00
mg NTG/in.^{2} patch	12.90	31.79	78.59
Dissolution[a]			
30 min			
(Av mg NTG released per 1.0 sq. in.)	0.66	1.59	3.35
(Av % NTG released per 1.0 sq. in.)	5.11%	5.00%	4.26%
60 min	0.89	2.68	4.78
	6.89%	8.43%	6.08%
120 min	1.37	3.31	8.71
	10.62%	10.41%	11.08%
180 min	1.47	3.94	9.86
	11.39%	12.39%	12.54%

Note: First number of each entry = 30 min av. mg NTG released; percent = av. % NTG released.

[a] All analyses were performed on 1.0-in.^{2} patch.

Table 3
POLYMER MODIFICATION

Modifier	Mg NTG in patch	Dissolution mg released 0.5 hr
None	92	5.0
Tween 20	64	7.0
Glycerine	63	3.5
Squalene	67	6.2
Polyethylene	65	3.3
Triglyceride	51	6.7
Azone	31	3.3
M-Pyrol	41	2.5

C. Acute Dermal Toxicity in Rabbits

The purpose of this study was to evaluate the possible percutaneous toxicity of the referenced nitroglycerin (NTG) patch material.

Two groups of six in New Zealand white rabbits (three male, three female) each were used. One group received a placebo material as a control article. On the back of each rabbit

Table 4
COMPARATIVE DISSOLUTION STUDIES

Time	Hercon (1.0 in²)	Ciba (10 cm²)	Key (10 cm²)	Searle (8 cm²)
3-hr run				
30 min	5.18	0.64	8.35	4.20
Av mg NTG released per 1.0 in.²				
Av % NTG released per 1.0 in.²	7.1%	3.9%	25.3%	32.5%
2-hr run	10.07	1.64	18.90	6.64
	13.8%	10.1%	57.4%	51.4%
4-hr run	13.60	2.61	24.97	8.70
	18.6%	16.1%	75.9%	67.4%
6-hr run	16.35	3.71	27.50	9.86
	22.3%	23.0%	83.5%	76.4%
8-hr run	18.32	4.81	28.35	10.65
	25.0%	29.8%	86.1%	82.5%

Note: First number of each entry = 30 min av. mg NTG released per 1.0 in²; percent = av. % NTG released per in².

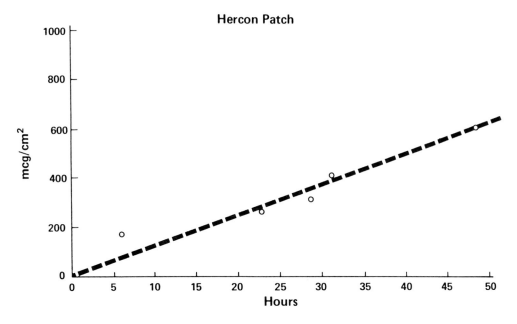

FIGURE 6.   Nitroglycerin penetration across female cadaver skin.

an area slightly larger than 240 cm² was clipped free of visible hair approximately 24 hr prior to application of the test material. Epidermal abrasions were made every 2 to 3 cm over the exposed area just prior to application of the test material.

A 240 cm² piece of test patch (approximately 1500 mg NTG-active; 0 mg NTG-placebo) was applied to the test site and occluded for a 24 hr exposure period.

The foam backing used in conjunction with this formulation was observed to cause erythema in all animals, when in contact with the skin. There was also some degree of discomfort encountered in each animal when the foam backing was removed from the skin.

No untoward toxic symptoms were noted at any time during the study.

Table 5
ANIMAL STUDIES: RABBIT

Product	Size (cm²)	mg NTG released per 24 hr	mg/cm²
Ciba	10.0	15.0	1.5
Hercon	6.45	14.5	2.25

Table 6
ANIMAL STUDIES: DOG

Product	Size (cm²)	mg NTG released per 24 hr	mg/cm²
Ciba	10.0	8.7	.87
Hercon	6.45	6.0	.93

D. Animal Dose Evaluation Study

A representative Hercon patch was tested on rabbits (New Zealand White) and dogs (Beagle) to determine skin permeation in vivo. Four groups of five animals each per species were used. The control groups had 48 hr exposures and the treatment groups 12, 24, and 48 hr exposures. The Ciba Transderm Nitro® 5 (10 cm²) and a Hercon test patch (6.45 cm²) were the test articles. The amount of nitroglycerin permeating through the skin was calculated by subtracting the mean postexposure assay for each patch. The results are shown in Tables 5 and 6 and indicate that the Ciba and the Hercon patches delivered equivalent amounts of nitroglycerin per unit surface area of skin.

V. BIOAVAILABILITY STUDY

A. Introduction

The objective of the study was to evaluate the systemic bioavailability of three Hercon topical nitroglycerin dosage forms as compared to a nitroglycerin ointment (Nitro-Bid®).

Sixteen healthy male subjects were administered, in a randomized order, four topical nitroglycerin dosage forms. The three transdermal patch delivery systems (O2M-A, O2M-B, and O2M-BM) were administered as a 124-mg single dose (two 10-cm² patches, each containing 62 mg nitroglycerin) on the subjects. The patches remained on the subject's chest for 72 hr. The ointment was administered as three 0.5 gm administrations (11 mg nitroglycerin every 8 hr) over a 24-hr period. The ointment was delivered by outlining a 50-cm² area on the subject's chest and evenly spreading the 0.5 gm ointment dose over this area. The 50-cm² application area was covered with a 75-cm² piece of aluminum foil and completely occluded with surgical tape. The three daily administrations of ointment were placed on different areas of the subject's chest. Serial blood (plasma) samples were collected for nitroglycerin analysis and Laser Doppler Velocimetry (LDV) measurements were taken for up to 24 hr after the first ointment application and 73 hr after the patch applications. The patches were removed 72 hr after application and the ointment dose was removed 8 hr after the third dose. The 72.5- and 73.0-hr blood samples were collected after removal of the patches.

Concentrations of nitroglycerin in plasma were determined with a gas chromatographic method employing a capillary column, an on-column injection system, programmed temperature gradient, and electron capture detection.

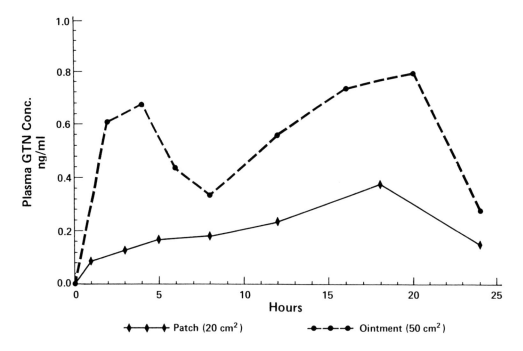

FIGURE 7.   NTG plasma results.

B. Results

The individual and mean plasma results of patch O2M-A are presented in Figure 7. The patch had a mean concentration maximum (C_{max}) of 0.381 ± 0.231 ng/ml at 18-hr postdrug. It produced nitroglycerin concentrations of above 0.1 ng/ml from 3- to 72-hr postdrug. The mean concentration of the 11 collection times to 72 hr is 0.176 ± 0.079 ng/ml. The O2M-A patch, the only one to be discussed in this presentation developed the highest nitroglycerin plasma levels of the three experimental patch products and had the lowest variability. This patch showed good skin adhesive properties throughout the 72 hr-application period.

The Nitro-Bid® ointment's mean and individual plasma levels with the outliers removed are also presented in Figure 2. The highest mean plasma concentration was after the third ointment dose (0.794 ± 0.441 ng/ml) at the 20-hr time point which was 4 hr after the last dose.

The 0- to 24-hr AUC relative bioavailability comparisons (normalized for surface area) indicated that patch O2M-A is 99.9% of the actual ointment 0- to 24-hr AUC value. These data indicate that patch O2M-A has adequate bioavailability when compared to the ointment. The mean concentration maximum (C_{max}), mean concentration and AUC values for the Hercon Patch O2M-A compare favorably to those published for the Ciba, Searle, and Key products.[7]

REFERENCES

1. **Bernstein, B. S., Kapoor, R., and Hyman, S.,** U.S. patent 4284444, 1981.
2. **Crank, J. and Park, G. S., Eds.,** *Diffusion in Polymers,* Academic Press, New York, 1968.
3. **Richards, R. W.,** The Permeability of Polymers to Gases, Vapors, and Liquids, ERDE Tech. Report 135, March 1973, Natl. Tech. Inf. Serv. AD-767, Washington, D.C., 627.
4. **Baker, R. W. and Longsdale, H. K.,** Membrane-controlled delivery systems, in Proceedings of Controlled Release Bioactive Materials Symposium, Cardarelli, N. F., Ed., University of Akron, Ohio, 1974, 40, 1.
5. **Crank, J.,** The Mathematics of Diffusion, Oxford University Press, London, 1975.
6. **Kydonieus, A. F.,** The effect of some variables on the controlled release of chemicals from polymeric membranes, in *Controlled Release Pesticides,* ACS Symp. Ser. 53, Scher, H. B., Ed., American Chemical Society, Washington, D.C., 1977, 152.
7. **Chien, Y. W.,** Logics of transdermal controlled drug administration, *Drug Dev. Ind. Pharm.,* 9(4), 497, 1983.

Chapter 12

TRANSDERMAL DRUG DELIVERY FROM HYDROPHILIC MATRIX MEMBRANES RESERVOIR SYSTEMS

Alan C. Hymes and David Rolf

TABLE OF CONTENTS

I. INTRODUCTION

The existing reservoir systems are polymeric matrix types except for the Alza-membrane system.[1-3] The matrix is an "open cell molecular sponge" wherein the polymers are the "sponge" held together by chain and cross-linking bonds. The fluid within the "sponge" is a plasticizer which contains the drug in a soluble and/or suspended state in a microspace suspended by the polymeric meshwork of linkages.

II. LECTEC MATRIX RESERVOIR

A new variation on existing polymeric transdermal delivery systems employs hydrophilic gel matrix membranes. It may contain one or a mixture of hydrogen bonding liquids, such as water, glycerine, propylene glycol, polyethylene glycol, etc. comprising from 40 to 70% of the total patch weight. Gellation agents employed always possess a high molecular weight and may include polysaccharides, such as karaya, algin, xanthan, guar, locust bean gum, and others and/or synthetic hydrophilic polymers, such as polyacrylamide, polyvinyl sulfonates, polyvinyl alcohol, polyacrylic acid, polyvinyl pyrrolidone, and others. The total amount of solids in a formulation can vary from 30 to 60% total weight. These formulations may also include aqueous emulsions of polymeric adhesives to improve the strength and tack of a drug patch. They will form gels at room temperature after a few hours, however, the rate of gellation is easily increased by heating. This provides a great deal of variability in the formulation since chemical characteristics can be modified by processing. The activity of a drug in a formulation can be adjusted by variation in the formula composition. This, in combination with drug concentration modification, allows one to control to some degree the rate of release of the drug from the patch.

Each matrix will have to be formulated for a specific drug and packaging of the matrix may also require much attention. For example, the great volatility of nitroglycerin makes it a unique drug requiring special packaging procedures. The drug molecule may have an affinity to the solvent and/or polymeric structure depending on the ionization structure of the polymer. Conversely, there may be no affinity to the matrix or an actual repulsion from the reservoir. Furthermore, all these forces can be significantly influenced by applying an electric current to the reservoir.

The mechanism of gelation of hydrogels is believed to be one of hydrogen bond rearrangement producing a stable cross-linked gel because all the patch components can be separated and recovered by chemical extractions. These materials usually exhibit a tendency to swell in high humidity conditions. The complex hydrogen bond network created by the hydration of the gelating agents with the liquids is, on a molecular level, fluxional. Since it is believed that no covalent bonds are formed during curing, the risk of irreversibly incorporating the drug into the gel matrix is minimized.

Characteristics of an Ideal Reservoir
1. Hold the drug in a stable reservoir
2. Have little or no affinity for the drug
3. Maintain structural integrity at high humidity and body temperature
4. Self-adhering
5. Reapplication to different skin sites
6. Nonirritating
7. Maintains good contact with skin
8. Simple construction and inexpensive to manufacture

III. SKIN DYNAMICS CONTROLLING ABSORPTION

The skin as a rate-controlling membrane is the most important part of a transdermal drug delivery system. Under certain conditions, the correlation of in vitro skin permeation test results with the corresponding in vivo results may be poor. In the LecTec system, the skin itself determines the limitation of the rate of diffusion from the reservoir to the systemic system.

The skin is a multilayered organ which has qualitative differences throughout the surface of the body. The cells next to the adipose tissue are in a layer called the stratum germinativum. This stratum is lined up like a fence, one cell thick, and is also called the basal cell layer. The next layer is the stratum malpighii which contains a number of cells (Prickle cells) piled on top of each other like styrofoam balls in a box. These cells migrate from the basal cell layer toward the surface.[4] The cells on the surface (stratum granulosum) are dehydrated and water is reabsorbed in to the lower layers.[5] The protective layer of "dead skin" is on the surface and is known as the stratum corneum.[4] This layer is the primary layer which causes electrical impedance and acts as a diffusion barrier to drugs. When wet, this surface becomes hydrated increasing in volume by as much as 40%.[6] The LecTec hydrophilic reservoir wets the stratum corneum, and creates the good contact required for migration of medicaments into the skin. There is evidence to suggest that barrier characteristics may be altered by changes in the formulation of the matrix reservoir.[7]

IV. SUMMARY

A semisolid state polymeric-matrix system has been described which functions both as a reservoir and a hydrophilic bridge to the skin simultaneously preparing the skin surface (stratum corneum) for drug penetration. It is easily removable and reapplied, and relatively inexpensive to manufacture.

Systemic transdermal delivery rates may be a function of the following:

1. The reservoir system
2. The reservoir-skin interface
3. The drug concentration in the aqueous phase within the skin
4. The capillary wash-out rate within the skin

REFERENCES

1. **Sved, S., McLean, W. M., and McGilveray, I. J.,** The influence of the method of application on pharmacokinetics of nitroglycerine from ointment in humans, *J. Pharm. Sci.,* 70, 1368, 1981.
2. **Chien, Y. W.,** Logic of Transdermal Controlled Drug Administrations, presented at Industrial Pharmaceutical R & D Symposium, Rutgers University, New Brunswick, N.J., January, 1982.
3. **Anon.,** *Medical World News,* November 23, 1981.
4. **Pinkus, H. and Mehregan, A. H.,** *A Guide to Dermatohistopathology,* 3rd ed., Appleton-Century-Crofts, New York, 1981, chap. 1.
5. **Baden, H. P. and Freedberg, I. M.,** Biosynthesis and structure of epidermal hair root and nail proteins, *Dermatology in General Medicine,* 2nd ed., McGraw-Hill, New York, 1979, chap. 8.
6. **Zellickson, A. S., Zellickson, B. M., and Zellickson, B. D.,** Measurements by transmission electron microscopy of dry skin before and after application of a moisturizing cream, *Am. J. Dermatopathology,* 4.3, June 1982.
7. **Bowman, David W.,** *Effect of Surfactants on Skin Permaeability* RXPO Short Course Session, "Modern Concepts in Totally Applied Drugs and Delivery Systems", June 18, 1984, New York.
8. **Freinkel, R. K.,** Lipids of the skin, *Dermatology in General Medicine,* 2nd ed., McGraw-Hill, New York, 1979, chap. 12.

Chapter 13

ULTRAMICROPOROUS CELLULOSE TRIACETATE MEMBRANES FOR TRANSDERMAL DRUG DELIVERY

Arthur S. Obermayer

TABLE OF CONTENTS

ABSTRACT

The transdermal drug delivery systems developed at Moleculon are based on Poroplastic® membranes or films. There are a number of different types of devices which use these membranes and the Poroplastic® membrane itself is compatible with essentially all drugs and vehicles. In practice, Poroplastic® systems are sufficiently versatile so that typical limitations related to the materials of construction and design of transdermal patches are virtually eliminated, and attention can be focused on preparing a formulation that will allow drugs to penetrate through the skin at an appropriate rate.

I. CHARACTERISTICS OF POROPLASTIC® MEMBRANES

Poroplastic® membranes are an open-cell ultramicroporous form of cellulose triacetate. The base polymer was first made in 1865[1] and has a long history of application to commercial products. Its biocompatibility and lack of skin sensitivity is exemplified by its common use as a kidney dialysis membrane in direct contact with blood and its use in Arnel® triacetate fabrics in continuous contact with the skin. All toxicological studies[2] have shown it to be inert and safe for oral and topical use. Cellulose triacetate itself is stable at temperatures in excess of 200°C and within the pH range of biological interest. It is compatible with essentially all vehicles that might be considered for medical applications and can be sterilized with radiation or ethylene oxide.

The Poroplastic® membrane itself is made by a patented process[3] involving low-temperature water coagulation of a solution of cellulose triacetate in organic acid. The initial product can be produced in a controlled manner so as to contain anywhere from 70 to 98% water by weight,[4] and this initial weight percent of water defines the "MA-number" used to identify different grades of Poroplastic® membranes. The water can subsequently be exchanged for almost any other liquid or solution by a simple diffusional exchange process. Thus, a Poroplastic® membrane is often referred to as "a solid composed mostly of liquid". The mechanical properties of water- and mineral oil-filled Poroplastic® membranes are compared in Table 1. The cellulose triacetate matrix is generally chemically inert to the drugs and solvents contained in it. Because it holds liquid solely by capillary action, it can also be described as "a molecular sponge". However, the pores are perhaps a million times smaller than those of an ordinary sponge, i.e., of molecular dimensions. It is, therefore, transparent and the capillary action retaining the liquid within the porous structure is very much stronger than in an ordinary sponge.

A. Characteristic Pore Dimensions

The characteristic pore dimensions can be inferred from measurements of molecular weight cutoff in the filtration of globular proteins of well-defined sizes as shown in Table 2.[5] A direct correlation between the water content of a Poroplastic® membrane and its molecular weight cutoff can be observed and is shown in Figure 1.[6] The molecular weight cutoff can then be used to estimate a characteristic pore diameter. The pores have reasonably broad size distribution, probably with a preponderance below the characteristic diameter.

B. Diffusive Permeability

A characteristic of particular importance for transdermal drug delivery through a Poroplastic® membrane is its diffusive permeability which can be varied over a broad range. It is one of the few essentially solid materials whose diffusive permeability in the unmodified form, as shown in Table 3,[7] is almost as high as is normally expected for liquids, i.e., area corrected diffusion coefficients are 1/4 to 1/2 what they would be for the pure liquid. This means that very rapid equilibration can be established throughout the interior of the membrane

Table 1
PROPERTIES OF POROPLASTIC® FILM

Property	Aqueous MA-70	Aqueous MA-92	Oil MA-70	Oil MA-92
Composition				
Resin, %	30	8	30	8
Water, %	70	92	—	—
Mineral oil, %	—	—	70	92
Specific gravity	1.09	1.02	1.01	0.91
Tensile strength, psi	1,300	175	2,300	400
Elongation at break, %	44	20	41	32
Tensile strength after drying, psi	2,600	550	—	—
Elastic modulus, psi	21,000	200	41,000	3,400
Elongation at elastic limit, %	2.4	4.0	2.4	3.1

Table 2
RETENTION CHARACTERISTICS OF POROPLASTIC® FILM

Solute	Molecular weight	% Retention at 30 psi on 4-mil films			
		MA-70	MA-85	MA-92	MA-92.5
Phenylalanine	165	0	0	0	0
Sucrose	342	0	0	0	0
Vitamin B-12	1,355	70	0	0	0
Inulin	5,200	—	10	0	0
Cytochrome C	12,400	>99	87	7	0
β-Lactoglobulin	35,000	>99	—	—	0
Hemoglobin	64,000	>99	97	—	0
Albumin (bovine)	67,000	>99	95	25	0
γ-Globulin	153,000	>99	>99	>98	0
Apoferritin	480,000	>99	>99	>99	42
Blue Dextran 2000	2,000,000	>99	>99	>99	93
Apparent pore diameter (Å)		14	25	60	>200
Apparent pore diameter (μ)		0.0014	0.0025	0.006	>0.02
Water content by weight (%)		70	85	92	97.5

which provides much flexibility in patch design. Additionally, due to this rapid equilibration, Poroplastic® membranes can be manufactured and loaded with a drug using a continuous process resulting in a high product throughout. For room temperature and low viscosity liquids, the equilibration times can be roughly approximated according to the following equation: $t_{90\%} = T^2$, where $t_{90\%}$ is the time in seconds for 90% equilibration and T is the thickness of the membrane in mils (0.001 in.). Thus, for a 10-mil thick membrane, 90% equilibration should be achieved in about 100 sec. This approximation is helpful in determining the minimum time for equilibration, but to be safe, much longer times should be used.

II. POROPLASTIC TRANSDERMAL SYSTEMS

A. Kinetic Alternatives

There are two very different conditions for which transdermal patches can be designed. In the first case, the process for drug penetration out of a patch to the surface of the skin is slower than its penetration through the skin. In the other case, the slower step involves

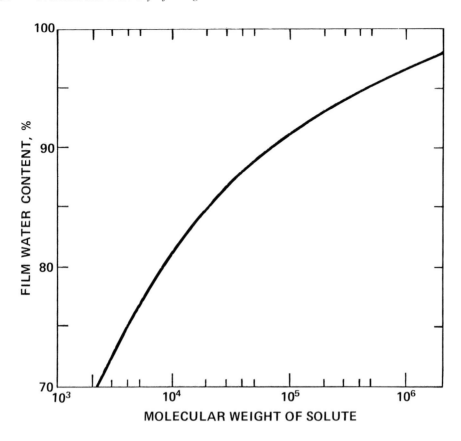

FIGURE 1.   Effect of water content on molecular weight cutoff (90% retention 0.004-in. film).

Table 3
DIFFUSIVE PERMEABILITY OF POROPLASTIC® MEMBRANE

Effect of Mol Wt on Diffusion for MA-85 Membrane

Solute (%)	Mol wt	Transport method	Diffusion coefficient (cm²/sec × 10⁻⁶)
0.3 NaCl	58	Film, 4 mil	4.9
0.2 Urea	60	Hollow fiber	1.6
2.0 Ionic chemical	400	Film, 4 mil	1.9
0.005 Vitamin B-12	1355	Hollow fiber	0.25

Effect of Membrane Water Content on Diffusion for 2% Ionic Chemical with Mol Wt of 400 to 4 mil film at 32°C

Poroplastic® Film	Flux (mg/cm²/sec)	Diffusion coefficient (cm²/sec × 10⁻⁶)
MA-92 film	0.00411	2.1
MA-85 film	0.00378	1.9
MA-70 film	0.00291	1.4
Average area corrected diffusion coefficient		2.2

drug penetration through the skin itself. The overall rate of any kinetic process can only be as fast as the slowest step, i.e., the rate-determining step. More rapid steps before or after the rate-determining step have little influence on the overall rate of the process. For example, rates of penetration through the epidermal and dermal layers will be unimportant for most drugs, because they are much more rapid than penetration through the outer stratum corneum layer. Similarly, when the slower or rate-determining step lies within the patch itself, the behavior of the skin is relatively unimportant.

B. Patch Rate Determining

For highly potent, rapidly penetrating drugs, it is possible to design patches in which the rate control is within the patch itself. Such systems potentially allow for accurate metering of drug delivery independent of variations in skin permeation characteristics between different individuals. In practice, however, relatively few drugs have sufficient potency and penetration rates to make this approach applicable. When it is feasible, the patch must be designed to provide only very slow diffusive drug delivery.

In Poroplastic® membranes, the intrinsic diffusive permeability is quite high but there are a number of methods for reducing permeability so as to make the membrane itself rate controlling. For example, the diffusive permeability can be reduced by:

1. Reducing the liquid content and partially collapsing the pores, thereby reducing the permeability, which can ultimately be made to approach the low diffusivity typical of pure cellulose triacetate
2. Providing a thin, low permeability skin on the surface of the Poroplastic® membrane similar to the thin skin on an asymetric reverse osmosis or ultrafiltration membrane[8]
3. Loading the Poroplastic® membrane with a solvent in which the drug has only slight solubility, thereby reducing the concentration dependent driving force for diffusion

C. Skin Rate Determining

It is much more common for the rate of drug penetration through the stratum corneum layer of the skin to be slow compared with processes that take place within the patch itself. Under these conditions, the patch should be designed so that the optimal drug composition is always available at the patch/skin interface. For Poroplastic® membranes, because of their high intrinsic diffusive permeability, rapid equilibration of the dissolved drug takes place throughout the membrane. Thus, the drug concentration at the patch/skin interface can remain constant as well as the resulting rate of release.

It is possible to treat the kinetics of this process semiquantitatively in the following manner. For a diffusive membrane of fixed thickness, the rate of penetration of any solute can be expressed by some penetration constant k multiplied by the thermodynamic activity a on the more concentrated side of the membrane. While this is strictly true only when the exit activity is virtually zero and diffusive equilibrium has been attained, it represents a firm upper bound for transport through a membrane which has not recently been exposed to any input activity in excess of a; the real rate may be slower, but not faster.

Now consider the case where the penetration constant of some drug through the skin, k_s, is much less than that for the same drug through the Poroplastic® membrane acting to supply a drug to the skin, k_m. Under these conditions of thermodynamic equilibrium within the membrane, diffusive processes within the membrane will be much too fast to be significantly perturbed by the loss of drug, and the drug concentration will remain almost uniform at some value c_m throughout the membrane. The thermodynamic activity of the drug can then be closely approximated by the ratio of its concentration to the saturated concentration, c_{sat}, for the drug in the solvent system being used. That activity, however, must then be the same as the drug activity at the surface of the skin, which serves to drive the diffusion process through the skin. Thus, in the case where $k_m \gg k_s$ one finds that

Penetration Rate $=$

$$R_p = k_s \cdot a = k_s \cdot \frac{c_m}{c_{sat}} \qquad (1)$$

D. Poroplastic® Patch Design

Poroplastic® patches have the appearance of an adhesive bandage and are fabricated by methods commonly used for such bandages. There are three alternative designs which can be used for the active component of the patch. The designs are adaptable to the conditions where either the patch or the skin is rate controlling. Figure 2 depicts each of these designs with a theoretical delivery profile.

1. **Simple Monolithic System** — The drug is incorporated directly into the Poroplastic® membrane in soluble form to be released slowly through the skin. The drug delivery rate follows Fick's laws. As the membrane is depleted of the drug, the concentration gradient decreases and the corresponding rate of penetration decreases with time. This system is inexpensive to manufacture and is relatively easy to adapt for most drug compounds.

2. **Distinct Reservoir System** — The drug is incorporated in a concentrated solution or suspended form behind a Poroplastic® membrane, providing a reservoir of drug. As drug transfers from the membrane to the skin, it is replaced rapidly by fresh drug from the reservoir. The drug is often released at a constant, time-independent rate for the life of the system. This system is more difficult and expensive to manufacture than the monolithic systems but it is more versatile.

3. **Zero Order Monolithic System** — The drug is incorporated as precipitated particles within the same layer of membrane that is in contact with the skin. It acts as a dispersed reservoir system in that each precipitated particle is in fact a small reservoir. The precipitated particles dissolve on demand to maintain a saturated drug solution. The very high diffusive permeability of the drug within Poroplastic® membranes allows the drug from the interior of the membrane to rapidly replace that which has left the surface and gone into the skin. Thus, saturation concentrations at the skin surface, and constant delivery rates are assured. Where applicable, this system combines the performance advantages of the distinct reservoir system with the manufacturing ease and safety of the simple monolithic system.

III. PRODUCTION BY FILM CASTING, DIFFUSIONAL EXCHANGE PROCESS

The manufacture of Poroplastic® membrane loaded with the appropriate drug composition for transdermal delivery can take place in a single continuous unit operation under mild conditions. A uniform thickness of a viscous cellulose triacetate solution is cast or coated onto a continuous web by a process similar to that used to make vinyl coated fabric. Then, the solution is coagulated and washed in a series of water baths. The details of the next steps in the process depend on the formulation of the drug to be introduced but generally it involves passing the already formed membrane through a series of exchange baths to convert to the proper solvent, introduce the drug and, where desirable, form a precipitate. Finally, the Poroplastic® membrane is wound up on a core at least one foot wide and hundreds of feet long. This type of process can produce uniform products thereby simplifying quality control procedures. The drug itself is subject only to mild conditions which can be important

POROPLASTIC® DRUG DELIVERY SYSTEMS

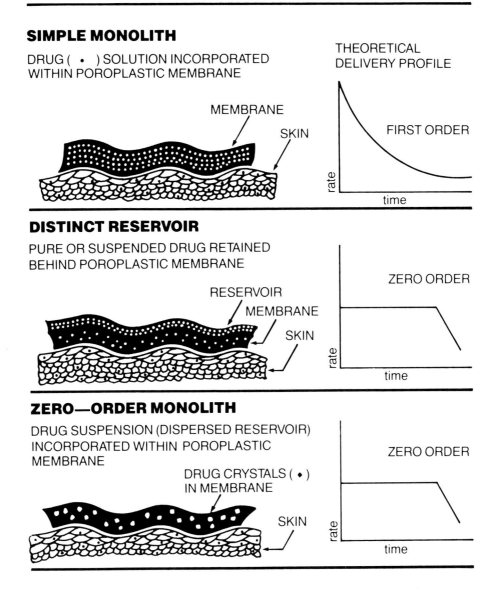

SIMPLE MONOLITH

DRUG (•) SOLUTION INCORPORATED
WITHIN POROPLASTIC MEMBRANE

THEORETICAL
DELIVERY PROFILE

MEMBRANE
SKIN
FIRST ORDER
rate
time

DISTINCT RESERVOIR

PURE OR SUSPENDED DRUG RETAINED
BEHIND POROPLASTIC MEMBRANE

ZERO ORDER

RESERVOIR
MEMBRANE
SKIN
rate
time

ZERO—ORDER MONOLITH

DRUG SUSPENSION (DISPERSED RESERVOIR)
INCORPORATED WITHIN POROPLASTIC
MEMBRANE

ZERO ORDER

DRUG CRYSTALS (•)
IN MEMBRANE
SKIN
rate
time

FIGURE 2. Examples of alternative approaches from drug delivery through Poroplastic® membranes.

for sensitive or unstable drugs. The diffusional exchange process is normally carried out at room temperature and does not require any catalysts, unusual pH, or solvents. It is a rapid process because of the very high diffusive permeability of the Poroplastic® membrane, i.e., for a typical 10-mil film, approximately 90% of the exchange will take place in 100 sec and 99% in 200 sec. Thus, for a line speed of 10 ft/min a liquid contact path length in the exchange bath of 17 ft would be required in order to get a 90% exchange. A roll of membrane, once produced, is then subject to standard bandage making equipment which produces the finished product patch. Standard bandage fabrication utilizes rolls of various components which are slit and cut to size and bonded to each other in the proper layered sequence. The Poroplastic® membrane essentially replaces the gauze in a typical adhesive bandage.

IV. FORMULATION AND APPLICATION

In Poroplastic® patches, there is usually no specific chemical interaction between the drug or its vehicle and the cellulose triacetate matrix. Since the Poroplastic® membrane acts as an inert molecular sponge, it can be loaded with just about any drug solution or suspension and the release kinetics will be independent of the effect of the matrix on the drug. This means that the key factor in controlling release rates is the formulation of the drug and vehicle that is to be put into the Poroplastic® membrane. In order for a drug to be a realistic candidate for transdermal delivery, it should be nonionic and of low molecular weight and have some solubility in water, but be even more soluble in lipids.

In experimental testing, the performance of different drugs, formulations, and patch designs are compared by normalizing data to the same active patch area in contact with the skin. The amount of drug delivered is directly proportional to the area of skin; thus, as long as the dimensions of the patch are kept within reasonable limits for market acceptance (typically under 25 cm^2), the total delivery can be increased by increasing area. In a similar manner, when the thickness of a patch is increased, it usually results in a proportionally larger reservoir and a proportional increase in the duration of drug delivery. In order to achieve maximum product elegance and fabrication ease, the preferred membrane thickness is approximately 0.05 cm.

It is the degree of saturation or thermodynamic activity of the drug in solution in the patch that determines the partitioning of the drug, i.e., the transference of drug from the patch to the surface of the skin. For rapid penetration through the skin, formulations which utilize saturated drug solutions are more effective. Note that it is the degree of saturation and not the concentration per se of drug that is the critical parameter.

Another approach to increasing penetration rates is to alter the character of the stratum corneum so that the rate constant for skin penetration is increased. This can be accomplished by means of various penetration aids.[9] Using such additives has proven to be effective with a number of Poroplastic® formulations.

At Moleculon, many different drug products have been evaluated in vitro and in vivo for transdermal delivery. These include such drugs as nitroglycerin, isosorbide dinitrate, phenylpropanolamine, chlorpheniramine, and triethanolamine salicylate as well as a large number of proprietary drugs. A variety of vehicles have also been utilized ranging from polyethylene glycol, water, and alcohols to aliphatic esters, mineral oil, and silicone oil.

The evaluation of drugs at Moleculon usually starts with a review of existing pharmacokinetic and physical chemical data to determine whether a particular drug is appropriate for in vitro testing. Drug candidates with acceptable profiles must then be formulated to provide acceptable therapeutic blood levels without causing irritation. These formulations are tested in micro-flow cells[10] of modified design using automatic sample collectors to allow regular sampling over a 24- to 72-hr period. Typically 28 cells are run at a time utilizing small sections from the same piece of freshly excised human skin recovered in the course of reduction mammoplasty procedures. Where practical radiotracer forms of the active drug are used, and penetration rate measurements are made with a liquid scintillation counter. The results of these measurements are fed directly into a microcomputer which provides plots of drug penetration rate vs. time. This is followed, if necessary, by skin irritation and blood level tests on animals in preparation for human clinical studies. For skin irritation tests, rabbits are normally used. Blood level tests for bioequivalence are most conveniently carried out using hairless mice. When a number of large blood samples are required, a larger animal must be used. Pigskin most closely simulates human skin, but is an expensive animal to use. In our experience, animal studies are of limited value because no animal skin bears a close resemblance to human skin. Thus, we eliminate animal studies where practical.

The versatility, adaptability, and convenience of Poroplastic® transdermal systems have made them increasingly attractive to major pharmaceutical companies. In the years ahead, it is expected that they will be utilized for the controlled delivery of many drugs.

REFERENCES

1. **Schutzenberger and Naudin,** *Z. Chem.,* 264, 1869.
2. **Nichols, L. D.,** Process of Preparing Gelled Cellulose Triacetate Products and the Products Produced Thereby, U.S. Patent 3,846,404.
3. Moleculon Research Corporation internal document on Poroplastic® toxicology. References on Toxicity of Cellulose Triacetate Membranes, Cambridge, Mass.
4. **Obermayer, A. S. and Nichols, L. D.,** Controlled release from ultramicroporous cellulose triacetate, ACS Symposium Series No. 33, 1976, 303.
5. **Obermayer, A. S. and Nichols, L. D.,** Controlled release from ultramicroporous cellulose triacetate, ACS Symposium Series No. 33, 1976, 305.
6. **Obermayer, A. S.,** in *Controlled Release Technologies; Methods, Theory, and Applications,* Kydonieus, A. F., Ed., CRC Press, Boca Raton, Fla., 1980, 242.
7. **Obermayer, A. S.,** in *Controlled Release Technologies: Methods, Theory, and Applications,* Kydonieus, A. F., Ed., CRC Press, Boca Raton, Fla., 1980, 243.
8. **Obermayer, A. S., Nichols, L. D., Allen, M. B., and Caron, R. P.,** Development of an Ultra-Thin-Skinned Reverse Osmosis Membrane Using Homogeneous POROPLASTIC® Film as the Ultramicroporous Substrate, Final Report, U.S. Department of Interior, Office of Water Research and Technology, Washington, D.C., 1981.
9. **Rajadhyaksha, V.,** *Controlled Release Transdermal Drug Delivery,* Kydonieus, A. F. and Berner, B., Eds., CRC Press, Boca Raton, Fla., 1984, chap 3.
10. **Bronaugh, R. L. and Stewart, R. F.,** Methods for in vitro percutaneous absorption studies. IV. The flow-through diffusion cell, *J. Pharm. Sci.,* 74, 64, 1985.

Chapter 14

DEVICES FOR MACROMOLECULES

Dean S. T. Hsieh

TABLE OF CONTENTS

I. INTRODUCTION

Drug depots which are either matrices, reservoirs, or hybrids of the two are essential components of transdermal drug delivery devices. So far, all Food and Drug Administration approved transdermal patches contain drugs with a molecular weight of below 320 daltons, such as nitroglycerin (mol wt 227), scopolamine (mol wt 303), estradiol (mol wt 312), and clonidine (mol wt 230). No transdermal patches containing macromolecules have yet been developed. It is still questionable whether polar compounds and/or high molecular weight compounds can permeate the skin. On one hand, fundamental understanding of the transdermal delivery of low molecular weight and nonpolar drugs is progressing rapidly. On the other hand, studies of controlled delivery of macromolecules from polymers are still in their infancy. Advances in both areas will provide clues to the feasibility of transdermal administration of macromolecules. This chapter summarizes the advances made in the fabrication of devices for the controlled delivery of macromolecules* from synthetic polymers, such as ethylene vinyl acetate copolymers and silicone elastomers. Detailed procedures for the preparation of devices for macromolecules may be obtained from the cited original research articles.

II. CONTROLLED RELEASE OF MACROMOLECULES FROM POLYMERS

There are three types of delivery vehicles which provide controlled release of macromolecules from polymers: (1) injectable microspheres, (2) depot-forming injectable liquid formulations, and (3) subdermal implants.

A. Injectable Microspheres

Microspheres can be prepared by a standard phase-separation or water-in-oil emulsion technique. In principle, active agents such as insulin[2] and analogs of LHRH[3] are "microencapsulated" in an envelope of biodegradable polymers. The biodegradable polymers used include polylactic/glycolic acid copolymer,[3] albumin,[4] crystallized carbohydrate,[5] hydrogels,[6] and polyanhydride.[7] The sizes of the resultant microspheres prepared with the phase separation method (or coacervation) are in the range of 2 to 5000 μm. To be injected with a hypodermic syringe, the microspheres should be below a few hundred micrometers (μm). The duration of the release of macromolecules from microspheres can last from 14 days, for the release of insulin to normalize blood glucose in diabetic rats,[2] to 40 days, for LHRH analog release to suppress estrus in rats.[3] This system is intended for parenteral administration of macromolecules, including intravenous (i.v.), intramuscular (i.m.), and subcutaneous (s.c.) injections.

B. Depot-Forming Injectable Systems

Alginate is a heterogeneous linear block copolymer of D-mannuronic acid and L-gluronic acid with 1,4-linkages; it has one free carboxylic and two free hydroxyl groups per uronic acid residue. Alginate as a sodium salt is soluble in water, but as a calcium salt it is insoluble. Due to this property, the preparation of calcium alginate gels for use in a sustained release delivery system is a very simple process. When droplets of sodium alginate solution containing bovine serum albumin are added to a solution of calcium chloride, stable gel beads are formed.[34]

---

* Therapeutic macromolecules which can be incorporated into polymeric devices include hormones, enzymes, biologically active peptides, growth hormones, interferon, mucoproteins, lipoproteins, nucleic acid, carbohydrates, monoclonal antibodies, and other biological products. Due to advances in genetic engineering, thousands of these therapeutic macromolecules may be mass-produced for clinical use.[1]

In 1950, D. Slavin used calcium alginate as an antigen depot for the production of antisera in rabbits. The rationale of the system was to condition the reticuloendothelial system, over a period of 3 weeks to a month, to the reception of continuous small doses of antigen, which were released from the alginate as the latter was absorbed. This was to be followed by i.v. inoculations of tolerable doses of the same antigen, so as to flood the reticuloendothelial system and thereby increase antibody production. This was accomplished by an i.p. inoculation of a 1.0 mℓ concentrate of culture emulsified in 4.0 mℓ of 5% sodium alginate, followed immediately by massage and the inoculation of 2.5 mℓ of 1% calcium chloride into the same site. The animal was left alone for 3 weeks to a month, and then given three intravenous inoculations of the same antigen at 4-day intervals. Slavin's final results showed antisera production to be as good as or better than that obtainable by conventional methods.[8]

C. Subdermal Implants

There are currently two approaches to this type of device. One is the use of biodegradable polymers, such as polylactic acid/glycolic acid copolymers, for the release of insulin in streptozotocin-diabetic rats,[9] and polyanhydrides, for the release of H^3-inulin in vitro.[10] The other is the use of nonbiodegradable polymers, such as ethylene vinyl acetate copolymers and silicone elastomer.

1. Ethylene Vinyl Acetate Copolymers

Ethylene vinyl acetate copolymers are white, odorless resins made of copolymerizing ethylene with vinyl acetate. Elvax®, a registered trademark of Du Pont which contains 40% vinyl acetate, is commonly used for drug delivery devices. A number of applications for these polymeric delivery devices for macromolecules have been explored. Some examples of their uses are

1. To prolong the release of insulin to maintain normoglycemia in diabetic rats for one month[11]
2. To provide a simple, safe and effective means of immunization by acting as a series of continuous minishots[12]
3. To create a concentration gradient for studying chemotaxis in biological systems[13]
4. To deliver informational macromolecules, such as tumor angiogenesis factor and growth factor, for bioassays[14]
5. To provide the drug delivery vehicle in studies of the development of corneal ulcers and in tests of the mechanism of vascular regression[15]

Furthermore, this polymer was used to prepare devices to deliver macromolecules at a magnetically modulated release rate.[16]

2. Silicone Elastomer

Silicone elastomers (polydimethylsiloxanes) have been used as drug delivery systems for the controlled administration of pharmaceuticals and veterinary drugs. The major advantages of using polydimethylsiloxanes in drug delivery are biocompatibility with body tissue and ease of fabrication. However, one of the disadvantages is the impermeability of ''polar'' compounds and the low permeability of water soluble drugs.[17] Recently, the feasibility of controlled release of macromolecules from silicone elastomers was explored. The kinetics of release, the biochemical activity, and a microstructural analysis of these macromolecules were reported.[18] Experiments which explore potential applications of this system are now being conducted.

III. FABRICATION PROCEDURES

When planning to fabricate devices for macromolecules, bear in mind the fact that macromolecules, in general, will not permeate polymer backbones. Therefore, the device must be designed in such a way that channels in the matrices are formed during the fabrication procedure in order to allow for the release of the macromolecules. There are two types of fabrication methods which have been employed to prepare synthetic polymer devices which allow for the sustained release of macromolecules. The solvent casting method is used to prepare devices made of ethylene vinyl acetate copolymers. The curing method is used to prepare devices made of silicone elastomers.

A. Solvent Casting

In the preparation of a sustained release polymeric delivery system for macromolecules using ethylene vinyl acetate copolymers (EVA), the polymer is dissolved in methylene chloride. The polymer solution is then mixed with "presieved" protein aggregates. Because both protein and polymers are long-chain macromolecules, a continuity restriction is imposed by their long-chain length. This causes problems in attempting to mix the two components together. The system is, therefore, incompatible from a thermodynamic standpoint, and the result is a cloudy dispersion. As shown in Figure 1, a polymer solution mixed with macromolecules (protein aggregates) quickly "gels" when cast on a glass mold placed on a block of dry ice at $-80°C$. After 2 days at $-20°C$ (under a mild vacuum), enough solvent evaporates to allow further drying at room temperature. This low temperature fabrication procedure[19] for the incorporation of proteins into polymeric matrices improves the reproducibility of the release kinetics when compared with the procedures first reported by Langer and Folkman.[20] The reproducibility of the release kinetics from polymer matrices prepared with the low temperature casting method is attributed to the following factors: (1) the presieving of protein aggregates lessens the heterogeniety of the irregular protein aggregates, (2) the rapid cooling step minimizes the settling of the protein aggregates, and (3) the low temperature drying step maintains the physical integrity of the matrices. The protein-polymer matrix shrinks about 40% because of the evaporation of the solvent.

Three fabrication parameters, loading, size of the aggregates, and coating affect the release kinetics significantly.[19] At the same loading, the release rate increases as particle size increases. Release rate increases caused by an increase in particle size may be a result of the formation of larger channels or pores in the polymer matrix. Similarly, increased loadings may provide simpler pathways (lower tortuosity) and greater porosity for diffusion, both of which would facilitate the movement of water into, and proteins out of, the matrix. Figures 2A and 2B show the effects of aggregate size and loading on the release profile of BSA from EVA matrices. The results seen in coating may be due to the fact that fewer macromolecules are on the matrix surface as well as the fact that the surface access of pores for channelled diffusion is decreased. The relationship between loading and the porosity of the matrices was investigated by Bawa.[21]

Four considerations in the design of devices for the release of macromolecules from ethylene vinyl acetate copolymers are

1. In some cases, the macromolecules must be delivered at a constant rate.
2. In some cases, the macromolecules must be delivered at a modulated release rate.
3. In some cases, the device must deliver a minute quantity of the sample.
4. The device should not shrink due to the loss of solvent.

1. Hemisphere-Shaped Devices[22]

The diffusion-controlled matrix device, because it is easily fabricated, has been one of

PREPARATION of SUSTAINED RELEASE POLYMERS

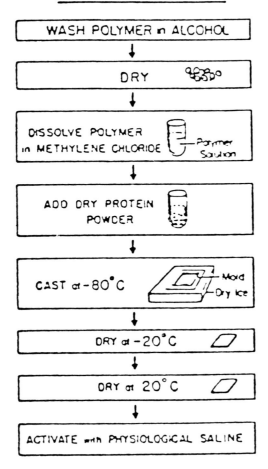

FIGURE 1. Flow diagram describing the procedures of the low temperature casting method for the preparation of systems for the sustained release of macromolecules. The alcohol wash was necessary to remove the impurities which cause inflammation of rabbit cornea.[19]

the most widely used drug delivery systems, but a disadvantage frequently cited is its inability to achieve zero-order release kinetics. Most matrix devices have been designed in the form of a rectangular slab, and it has been observed that the cumulative release of the drug is proportional to the square root of the elapsed time.[19] Mathematical analysis of different geometric designs of matrices[22,23] shows that the release rate of a hemisphere-shaped device (Figure 3) can be derived from Equation 1,

$$dQ/dt = 2\ C\ D\ a_i(R/R - a_i) \tag{1}$$

where a_i is the inner radius and R is the distance to the interface between the dissolved region (white area) and the dispersed zone (diagonal lines). The black area represents laminated regions through which release cannot occur. In examining Equation 1, it can be seen that $R - a_i$ becomes equal to R when $R \gg a_i$. Therefore,

$$dQ/dt = 2\ DC\ a_i \tag{2}$$

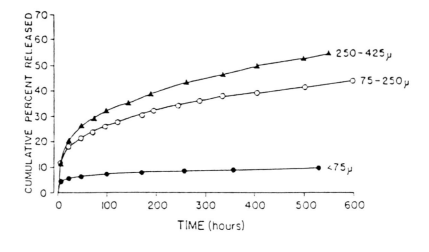

A

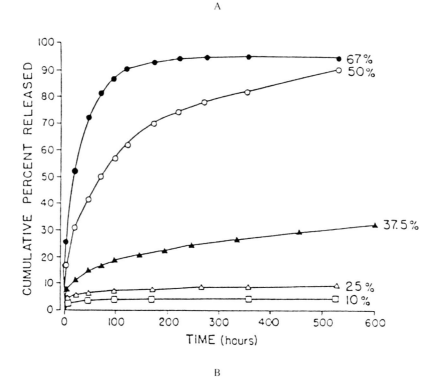

B

FIGURE 2. (A) Effect of size of the aggregates on the cumulative release of bovine serum albumin.[19] The loading is 25% w/w. The standard error of the mean of the cumulative release at each time point was within 10%. (B) Effect of protein content on the cumulative release of bovine serum albumin.[19] The particle size is less than 75 μm. The standard error of the mean of the cumulative release at each time point was within 10%.

Each of the terms in Equation 2 is a constant. Thus, for a hemisphere-shaped device with a small a_i, the release rate will be essentially constant.

It can be calculated that, for hemispheric devices designed so that the outer radius (a_o) is at least three times greater than the inner radius (a_i), zero-order kinetics will be achieved after a short burst and maintained for the duration of release.[23]

In an experiment to make hemisphere-shaped devices for the delivery of macromolecules,

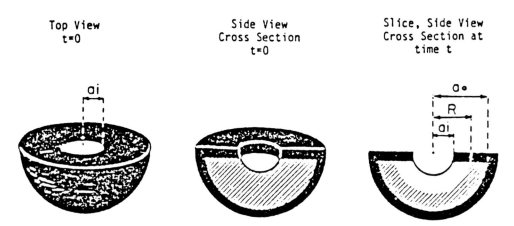

| Top View t=0 | Side View Cross Section t=0 | Slice, Side View Cross Section at time t |

FIGURE 3.   Schematic diagram of an inwardly releasing hemisphere, where a_o is the outer radius, a_i is the inner radius, and R is the distance of the interface between the dissolved region (white area) and the dispersed zone (slashed area). Black represents the laminated membrane through which release cannot occur.[22]

the solvent casting method of preparing polymer-macromolecular slabs[19] was used. The procedure is illustrated in Figure 4. In principle, two major steps are involved, the preparation of a hemisphere-shaped matrice and the coating of the devices followed by the opening of a cavity in the center of the flat surface. The first step is essentially the same as for preparing a slab, except that a hemispheric mold is used. Glass molds were made using the bottoms of test tubes. They were cut in the glass shop in the laboratory. The devices were coated with 20% EVA solution (containing no macromolecules) to form an impermeable barrier. The central cavity was formed by the insertion of a metal stick.

Figure 5 shows the release kinetics of albumin from the hemisphere-shaped device. A linear relationship between the cumulative percentage release and the time of release was observed for 60 days. The release rate was about 0.5 mg albumin per day. The fabrication parameters which affected the release kinetics are the size of the central cavity, loading, and aggregate size.

2. Magnetically Modulated Release Devices[16]

A unique problem central to the field of sustained release technology is that, so far, all vehicles have developed display drug releases which are either constant or which decay with time. There has been no way to change or modulate the release rate on demand, once release has commenced. In some circumstances, e.g., insulin delivery in diabetics, it would be useful to be able to obtain an increased dosage on demand. In one experiment, a sustained release system was developed which incorporated bovine serum albumin (BSA) as a model protein with magnetic steel beads in an ethylene vinyl acetate copolymer matrix. When exposed to aqueous medium, the polymer matrix released BSA slowly and continuously. Applying an oscillating magnetic field caused the release rate of BSA to increase by as much as 100%. Intervals of 6-hr periods of magnetic exposure and nonexposure were alternated over a 5-day period, resulting in corresponding increases and decreases in BSA release, establishing a pattern of modulated release.[16]

A flow sheet for the preparation of magnetic sustained-release polymers is shown in Figure 6. Several features pertinent to the preparation of magnetic devices are mentioned below:

1. The use of the low-temperature casting and drying method prevents migration of the albumin in the polymer matrices
2. The use of a three-step procedure can successfully embed the magnetic beads between two layers of a polymer-macromolecule mixture

FABRICATION of HEMISPHERE-SHAPED POLYMER MATRICES

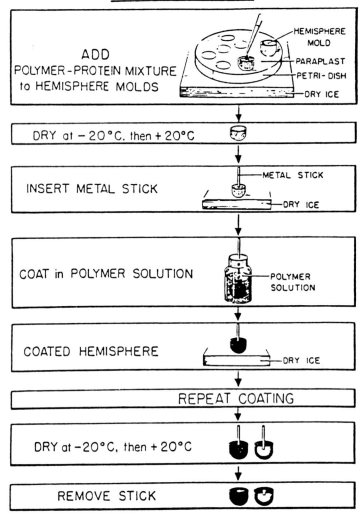

FIGURE 4. Flow sheet for preparing hemisphere-shaped devices for the release of macromolecules.[22]

3. Control of the casting time is critical to achieving vertical homogeneity of the matrix
4. The use of a specially designed loading device is very important in achieving horizontal homogeneity of the magnetic beads in the matrix
5. The magnetic beads used in the study were stainless steel beads, which are inert and biocompatible

Furthermore, a hemispheric magnetic device (Figure 7) was developed which combines an appropriate geometric design (to achieve a constant baseline release rate) with a magnetically modulated system (to obtain a burst of release upon triggering). The procedure for preparing the hemispheric magnetic system was adapted from earlier procedures and consists of four stages: casting, drying, coating, and opening a cavity (Figure 8). The rationale for selecting the procedures used, e.g., the low temperature casting, the three-step casting procedure, the drying procedure, and the desired geometric design, can be found in earlier

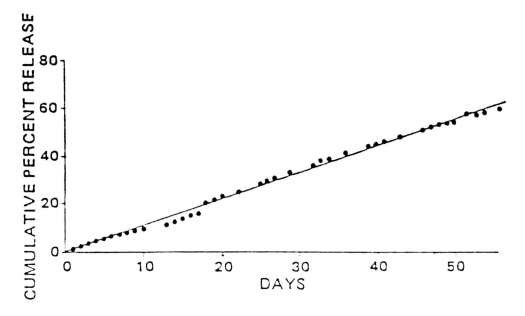

FIGURE 5. Cumulative release of bovine serum albumin versus time.[22] Standard error of the mean of the cumulative release at each time point was within 12%.

papers.[16,19,22] In the current study, two of those procedures were modified. A single magnetic ring, instead of many magnetic beads, was used because the magnetic domain, i.e., magnetic field strength, in this kind of magnetic ring is stronger than that of magnetic beads. Also, a paraplast platform was used to prevent the hemispheric glass molds from tilting.[24]

An example of the release of macromolecules from a hemispheric magnetic device is shown in Figure 9, indicating that the release of bovine serum albumin was modulated due to the magnetic device. The hemispheric magnetic devices were triggered for 5 hr followed by nontriggering for 19 hr. The cycle of triggering and nontriggering was repeated daily. There was a 29-fold increase in the quantity of BSA released during the period when the magnetic device was triggered, when compared with the nontriggering period. The major problems encountered in this design are irreproducibilities, both with respect to differences in release rates among different pellets within a given triggering period, and among the same pellets within different triggering periods.

3. Aqueous Dispersion Method[25]

It is not an easy task to prepare sustained release devices for minute quantities of a biologically active substance. Recently, the aqueous dispersion method was developed to incorporate minute quantities of samples such as interferon in EVA. The following procedure is used to produce these devices. An aqueous solution, mixed with a polymer solution, is cast at a low temperature, as it was in previous methods. The mixture is cooled to a temperature low enough to cause the water in the mixture to freeze. The frozen ice crystals create channels in the polymer device, which allow for the release of the active substance after both the water and the organic solvent are removed from the device. The organic solvent is removed by low temperature drying, and the water is removed by lyophilization.

This method provides improved drug release kinetics because freezing the water causes channel formation. The release rate can be adjusted by varying either the water:polymer ratio (Figure 10) or the concentration of the active substance (Figure 11). A typical example of the application of this method is the sustained release of interferon from EVA. The aqueous dispersion method is used with the many active substances which are available only as aqueous solutions or dispersions because it obviates the complicated and potentially destructive, e.g., denaturing, procedures for isolating and purifying the active substance.

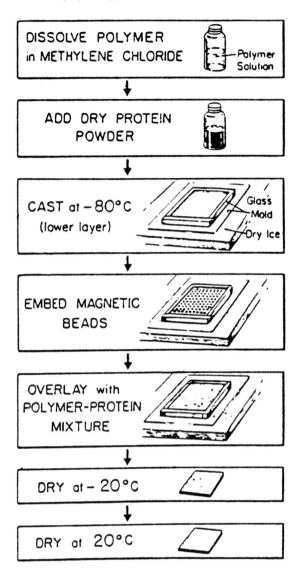

FIGURE 6.   Flow sheet for preparing magnetic sustained release systems for the delivery of macromolecules. A three-step casting procedure was used to achieve vertical homogeneity of magnetic beads, and a specially designed device was used to achieve horizontal homogeneity.[16]

4. Sintering Method[26,27]

Solvent casting always results in the shrinking of the finished devices. To minimize the problems of shrinkage and distortion of the matrix, the sintering technique is used to prepare devices for macromolecules such as insulin. The procedure consists of three stages: (1) pulverizing the ethylene vinyl acetate copolymers and agglomerating the insulin powder, (2) loading, heating, and compressing the polymer-insulin in a brass-mold, and (3) coating, drying, and then opening the cavity of the device.[26]

Two methods are employed in preparing EVA powders. In one, the EVA is dissolved in methylene chloride, followed by extrusion dropwise into liquid nitrogen. A mortar and pestle is used to grind the EVA particles into fine powder in the liquid nitrogen. The fine powder is then dried at a low temperature to allow the methylene chloride to evaporate.[26,27] The

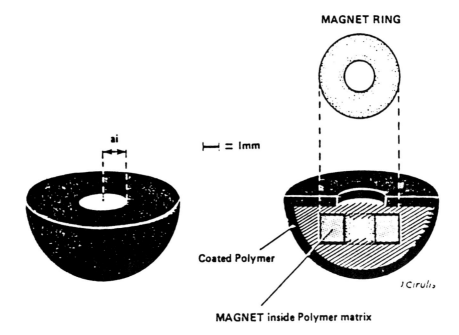

MAGNET RING

$\vdash\!\!-\!\!\dashv$ = 1mm

ai

Coated Polymer

J Cirulis

MAGNET inside Polymer matrix

FIGURE 7. Schematic diagram of a hemispheric magnetic device which delivers its content at a modulated release rate.[24] Black represents the laminated membrane through which release cannot occur. A magnetic ring was located in the center of the device. Drugs were released from the cavity on the flat face, shown by the white area of the device (left side).

other method involves precooling the EVA beads in liquid nitrogen, and then grinding them with an electric mill.[27]

It has been reported that formation pressure has a small effect on release kinetics. This effect tends to take place in the earliest stages of release, i.e., during the initial burst. The initial burst tends to decrease with increasing pressure. The release kinetics are also affected by the size and the age of the polymer particles.

This method is used to prepare hemispheric magnetic devices containing insulin. The blood glucose level (Figure 12) and the weight of diabetic rats (Figure 13) are normalized after implantation of this type of hemispheric magnetic device.[26]

B. Curing Method

As mentioned earlier, silicone elastomer is a very versatile polymer which has been used in drug delivery devices for the controlled administration of pharmaceuticals and veterinary drugs. Most applications have been limited to compounds of low molecular weight. However, devices have recently been fabricated for the delivery of macromolecules from silicone elastomers for long-term release.[18] The fabrication procedure is discussed in detail below.

1. Addition of Silicone Fluid

Silicone elastomer mixtures are made of medical grade silicone elastomers 382 and 360 (Dow Corning Co., Midland, Mich.) in the following proportions: 100:0, 80:20, and 50:50. After homogeneity of the mixture is achieved by mixing it with a lab-stirrer (Cole Parmer Instrument Co., Chicago, Ill.), BSA, chymotrypsin, pepsin, or insulin is slowly added to the elastomer mixture, followed by the addition of a drop of polymerizing catalyst M or stannous octoate (Dow Corning Co., Midland, Mich.). The ratio of the amount of catalyst to the polymer mixture is 1:10. The drug loading varies from 20 to 50% of the total weight. The disposable plastic beaker containing the mixture is then placed in a desiccator connected

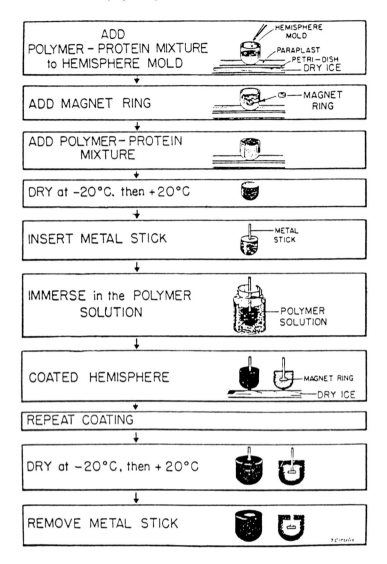

ADD
POLYMER – PROTEIN MIXTURE
to HEMISPHERE MOLD

HEMISPHERE
MOLD
PARAPLAST
PETRI – DISH
DRY ICE

ADD MAGNET RING

MAGNET
RING

ADD POLYMER – PROTEIN
MIXTURE

DRY at −20°C. then +20°C

INSERT METAL STICK

METAL
STICK

IMMERSE in the POLYMER
SOLUTION

POLYMER
SOLUTION

COATED HEMISPHERE

MAGNET RING
DRY ICE

REPEAT COATING

DRY at −20°C, then +20°C

REMOVE METAL STICK

FIGURE 8.   Flow sheet for preparing a hemispheric magnetic device.[24]

to a vaccum pump (Cole Parmer Instrument Co.) under 500 psi. The drug-polymer dispersion is then extruded into a section of Tygon® or Silastic® tubing (0.84 cm I.D. × 1.10 cm O.D.). The devices are cured overnight at room temperature in order to permit the completion of cross-linking. After the polymer is cured, the tubing is cut into pieces measuring 0.5 cm each. These are individually weighed and labeled. One end of the device is then coated with an impermeable coating, such as Silastic® medical adhesive silicone type A, leaving one end of the polymer exposed for protein release. The total surface area of the releasing plane of the matrices is 55.4 mm.

Using this procedure, macromolecule-silicone implants can deliver a variety of macromolecular compounds, such as bovine serum albumin, chymotrypsin, pepsin, and insulin. An experiment using BSA protein (aggregate size: 125 to 250 μm) at 35% loading, with silicone implants made of 80% silicone elastomer 382 and 20% silicone fluid 360 (Figure 14), resulted in long-term release of over 100 days. Control pellets which contained no BSA did not have any absorbance at UV 220 nm. The release rate calculated from the linearity of the curve was 128 μg/day. Figure 15 shows that at the same chymotrypsin loading,

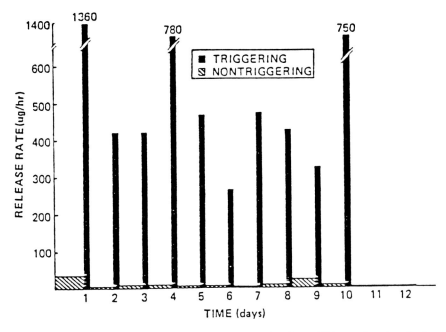

FIGURE 9.   Magnetic modulation of bovine serum albumin release.[24] Prior to triggering, the drug was allowed to leach from the device for 1 day. The devices were then triggered for 5 hr, which was followed by nontriggering for 19 hr. The cycle of triggering and nontriggering was repeated daily. (■) the quantity of BSA released during the magnetic triggering period, (▨) the quantity of BSA released during the nontriggering period.

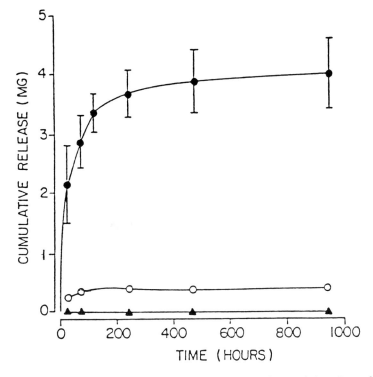

FIGURE 10.   Effect of the volume of protein solution on the cumulative release of bovine serum albumin from EVA pellets prepared with the aqueous dispersion method.[25] 5% (w/w) of BSA was mixed with 10 mℓ of 10% EVA solution. (▲) BSA dissolved in 0.1 mℓ of distilled water, (○) BSA dissolved in 0.2 mℓ of distilled water, (●) BSA dissolved in 0.3 mℓ of distilled water.

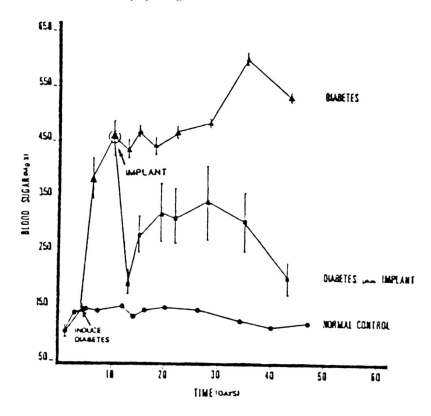

FIGURE 11. Effect of protein concentration on the cumulative release of bovine serum albumin from EVA pellets prepared with the aqueous dispersion method. The volume of aqueous-BSA solution is the same, except for the protein concentration.[25]

different silicone compositions resulted in different release rates of chymotrypsin. The matrices composed of 80% silicone elastomer 382 and 20% silicone elastomer 360 resulted in a greater release of proteins than from any other combination. The release rates were approximately 288 μg/day for an 80:20 combination, 220 μg/day for a 50:50 combination, and 190 μg/day for a 100:0 combination.

2. Addition of Co-Solvents

In the same experiment, additional preparations were made of medical silicone elastomer MDX 4-4210 (Dow Corning Co.) and co-solvents, such as glycerol, ethylene glycol, propylene glycol, and polyethylene glycol 400, in the following proportions: 100:0, 90:10, 80:20, and 70:30. The results indicated that when 20% w/w glycerol, ethylene glycol, propylene glycol, or polyethylene glycol 400 was added to BSA-silicone elastomer (MDX 4-4210) implants, the release fluxes of BSA, expressed as the total quantity of release over the square root of time ($Q/t^{1/2}$), were enhanced by 175, 108, 58, and 33%, respectively, when compared with those from virgin or placebo implants containing no additives (Figure 16 and Table 1). Note that the viscosity of silicone elastomer is closer to that of glycerol than to any other cosolvent (Table 1). Therefore, it is easier to mix silicone elastomer with glycerol than it is to mix any other combination. Insulin-containing implants made of silicone elastomer 382 and glycerol were implanted in diabetic rats, resulting in a reduction in hyperglycemia (unpublished data).

In another investigation, BSA-containing implants made of silicone elastomers 382 and 360 were prepared to investigate the effect of fabrication parameters, such as drug loading and aggregate size of proteins. Similar to devices made of EVA, the results showed that in

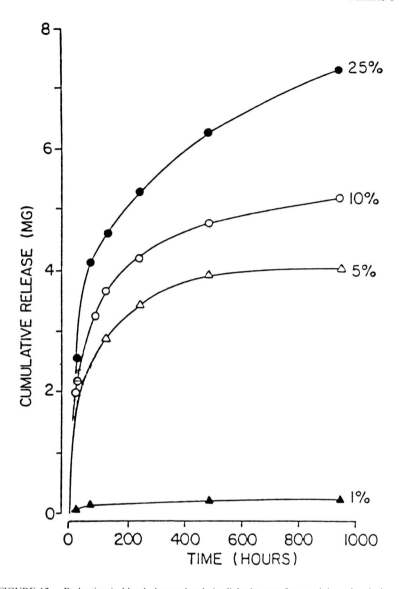

FIGURE 12. Reduction in blood glucose levels in diabetic rats after receiving a hemisphere magnetic device containing insulin. The control group consisted of diabetic rats which did not receive a device. A group of normal rats received neither the streptozotocin injection nor the device. Each group consisted of five rats.[26]

the macromolecule-silicone elastomer matrices, the higher the protein loading, the higher the release rate. However, at the same loading dose, there was no significant difference in release rates for protein aggregates of sizes in the range of 75 to 600 μm, except in the burst period ranging from 0 to 2 days.

These experiments with release kinetics have shown that silicone elastomers and macromolecules can be fabricated into matrix-type devices which deliver these macromolecules for over 100 days. Two features of the fabrication method developed in these studies are that the device is cured at room temperature and that no organic solvents are involved in the process.

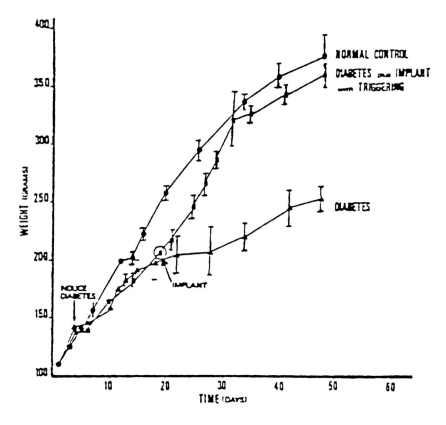

FIGURE 13.   Restoration of weight gain in diabetic rats after implantation of a hemispheric magnetic device containing insulin.[26]

IV. MICROSTRUCTURAL ANALYSIS AND MECHANISTIC INTERPRETATION

To study the potential release mechanisms of macromolecules from polymers, three types of silicone implants were examined by scanning electron microscopy. These implants were silicone elastomer-glycerol-BSA implants, both before and after complete leaching, and silicone elastomer-glycerol implants without proteins. For scanning electron microscopic analysis, silicone elastomer devices containing 35% BSA (aggregate size: 150 to 250 μm) were subjected to leaching. The silicone elastomer mixture was composed of 80% silicone elastomer MDX-4-4210, 10% catalyst, and 10% glycerol. When the leaching process had been completed, the devices were quickly frozen in Freon®, and then in liquid nitrogen. The samples were fractured, thawed in alcohol, and then subjected to critical-point drying procedures.[18] The samples were sputter-coated with 200 Å of gold-palladium, and then examined using an Emray® 1200 scanning electron microscope at 15 kV.

A microstructural analysis of the implants prepared with silicone elastomer-glycerol shows that glycerol vesicles are discretely dispersed throughout the matrix and apparently not interconnected with one another (Figure 17A). Before leaching, BSA aggregates were dispersed throughout the silicone elastomer-glycerol-BSA matrix, and no cavities were observed (Figure 17B). After complete leaching, the cavities were formed. The interconnected cavities were formed where the BSA aggregates had been (Figure 17C). Thus, this microscopic investigation of the polymeric matrices reveals the events that occur during the sustained release of macromolecules. When the polymer matrix is immersed in an aqueous medium, water diffuses into the matrix. Protein aggregates that are accessible to the aqueous medium,

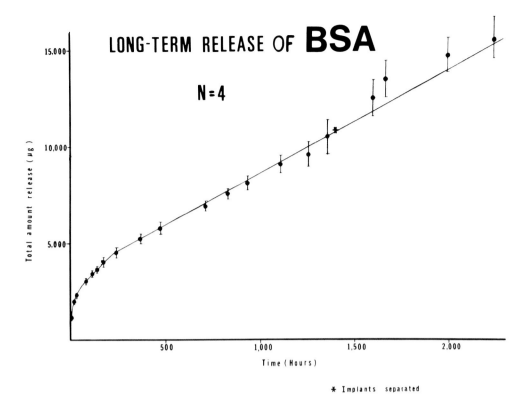

FIGURE 14. Long-term release of bovine serum albumin from silicone implants,[18] for 100 days. The protein loading was 35% and the aggregate size was 125 to 250 μm. The silicone implants were composed of 20% silicone fluid 360 and 80% silicone elastomer 382.

i.e., on the surface of the polymer matrix, are dissolved and diffused into the aqueous medium. This occurs within a short period of time. Water continues to diffuse into the polymer matrix and the protein aggregates absorb water. The protein aggregates inside the polymer matrix become a slurry within the voids of the matrix. At the same time, proteins diffuse into the medium. When all of the proteins have diffused out of the polymer matrix, the voids, which were previously occupied by protein aggregates, become empty spaces within the matrix.

In other words, progressive changes take place within the matrix in pore size and shape, in total porosity of the matrices, and in the size, shape, and concentration of the dispersed phase, i.e., protein. The diffusion of macromolecules throughout the porous polymer matrix is a function of position and time. This indicates that the system is in a transient state.

Equation 3 describes transient diffusion throughout a porous solid over time, as the variation of concentration within the pores.

$$\frac{\partial C_p}{\partial t} = D_{eff} \nabla^2 C_p \qquad (3)$$

Note the assumptions in the use of D_{eff} of (1) a single phase and (2) the invariance of D with position. The effective diffusion coefficient, D_{eff}, can be defined in the following formula:

$$D_{eff} = \frac{D_o k_r}{\tau} \qquad (4)$$

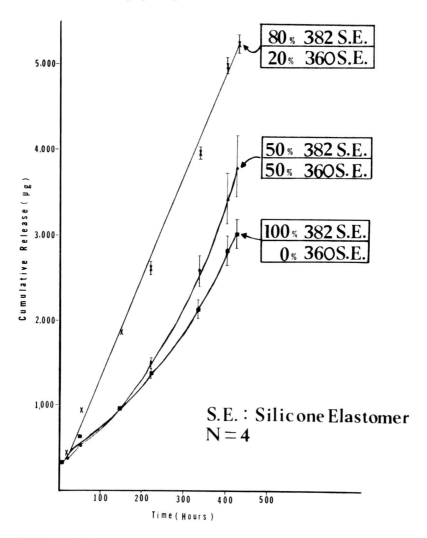

FIGURE 15.   Controlled release of chymotrypsin from silicone implants[18] prepared from various combinations of silicone fluid 360 and silicone elastomer 382. The enzyme loading was 30% w/w.

where D_o is bulk diffusivity; τ is the tortuosity; and k_r is the fractional reduction in diffusivity within the pore, which depends upon the value of λ ($= r_s/r_p$), the ratio of molecular diameter to pore diameter. When Colton et al.[28] studied restricted diffusion of macromolecules in porous beads, the following relationship was found

$$\log\left[\frac{\tau\, D_{eff}}{D_o}\right] = -2.0\,\lambda \qquad (5)$$

which can be applied to estimate the effective diffusion of certain compact and relatively rigid proteins.

V. LOGISTICS OF TRANSDERMAL DELIVERY OF MACROMOLECULES

The objective of this section is to present an opinion regarding the delivery of macromolecules by the transdermal delivery route. At the present time, the potential for the use

EFFECT OF CO-SOLVENTS

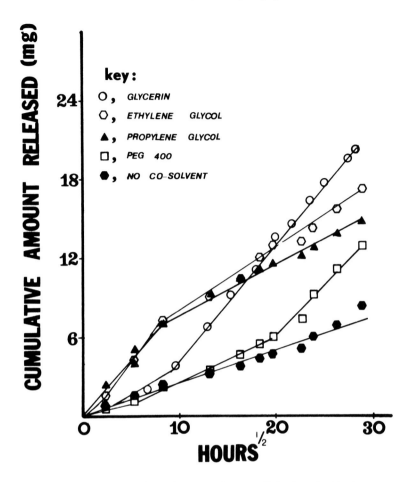

FIGURE 16.   The effect of co-solvents on the controlled released of bovine serum albumin from the silicone implants. The silicone polymer was composed of 70% MDX 4-4210 polymer base, 20% cosolvent, and 10% MDX 4-4210 catalyst.[18]

Table 1
EFFECT OF CO-SOLVENT ON RELEASE FLUXES OF BOVINE SERUM ALBUMIN FROM SILICONE IMPLANTS[a]

Co-solvent used in the implants[b]	Release flux (mg/cm^2/hr$^{1/2}$)	Relative[3] release rate (%)	Cumulative release (%)	Viscosity of co-solvent (cp)
Glycerol	2.65	275	33.8	1400
Ethylene glycol	1.96	208	29.1	2
Propylene glycol	1.14	158	25.8	50
PEG 400	0.96	133	22.1	101
No co-solvent	0.72	100	15.9	—

[a]   Protein used was bovine serum albumin whose molecular weight is 65,000.

[b]   Polymer base used in this study was silicone elastomer MDX 4-4210 whose viscosity is 800 cP.

[c]   Calculated from the ratio between release rates obtained from silicone implants containing co-solvent and those obtained from placebo implants without co-solvent.

SILICONE–GLYCEROL MATRIX

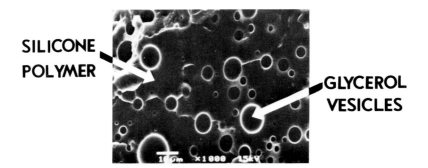

SILICONE POLYMER

GLYCEROL VESICLES

UNLEACHED

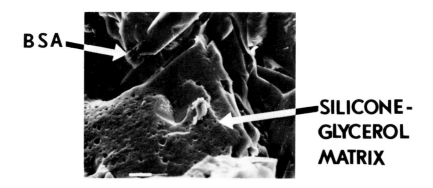

BSA

SILICONE– GLYCEROL MATRIX

COMPLETELY LEACHED

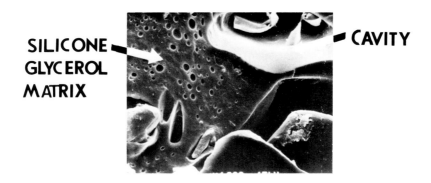

SILICONE GLYCEROL MATRIX

CAVITY

FIGURE 17.   (A) Scanning electron microscope (SEM) photograph of a silicone matrix containing glycerol.[18] The silicone polymer mixture was composed of 80% MDX 4-4210 polymer base, 10% glycerol, and 10% MDX 4-4210. (B) SEM photograph of a BSA-silicone elastomer-glycerol matrix before leaching.[18] BSA loading was 35% (w/w). The aggregate size was 150 to 250 μm. The silicone polymer mixture was the same as that in Figure 17A. (C) SEM photograph of a BSA-silicone elastomer-glycerol matrix after being completely leached.[18] The formulation was the same as that in Figure 17B.

Table 2
DIFFUSION COEFFICIENT AND MOLECULAR MASS
OF PROTEINS

Protein	Sedimentation coeff. S (sec)	Diffusion coeff. D (m²/sec)	Mol mass M	D/M$^{-1/3}$
Insulin	3.5×10^{-13}	8.2×10^{-11}	41,000	2.83×10^{-9}
Hemoglobin	4.4	6.3	67,000	2.56
Catalase	11.3	4.1	250,000	2.57
Urease	18.6	3.5	470,000	2.71

Note: The data was obtained at 20°C.[31]

of this means of delivery is not promising. However, the understanding of this delivery mode is improving and some investigators are focusing efforts in this area.

Dr. Albert Kligman, a dermatologist at the University of Pennsylvania School of Medicine, stated clearly that "the stratum corneum allows no substance to penetrate easily and allows all substances to enter slightly. With the sensitive methods now available, trace amounts can be detected."[29] He noted that, in his clinical experience, topically applied tuberculin, a filtrate obtained from titurated *Mycobacteria tuberculosis* containing 0.02 to 0.05 μg of purified protein derivative, has elicited a positive reaction in sensitive subjects. This implies that macromolecules can permeate the skin, although the extent to which permeation takes place is not known.

In contrast to this view, Dr. Jane Shaw of the Alza Corporation, in a rationale for the development of transdermal therapeutic systems, points out that, for transdermal applications, "suitable physico-chemical properties of a particular drug include stability, molecular weight less than 1000, melting point less than 200°F, solubility in both mineral oil and water greater than 1 mg/mℓ, and pH of 5 to 9 in a saturated aqueous solution."[30] Macromolecules may fail to satisfy most of these requirements, therefore, some authorities dismiss the possibility of transdermal administration of macromolecules.

Nonetheless, a logical approach is to look at the diffusion coefficient of macromolecules in aqueous solutions. Table 2 compiles the sedimentation coefficient, S, the diffusion coefficient, D, molecular mass, M (as determined by the ultracentrifuge), and the ratio of D/M$^{-1/3}$. Empirically, the relationship between the diffusion coefficient and the molecular mass of macromolecules can be expressed as:

$$D = K M^{-1/3} \qquad (6)$$

with a K value of 2.67×10^{-9} m²/sec. (The variation of K values among four proteins is within 5%.) For example, the diffusion coefficient of a peptide with molecular weight of 1000 is calculated to be 2.67×10^{-10} m²/sec, about a 30-fold increase when compared with insulin. Since a core of active site in protein molecules can be fragmented with the retention of its biological activity, and since most biologically active peptides are very potent requiring only a minute quantity to elicit a pharmacological response, the transdermal permeation of fragmented active sites of macromolecules may be possible.

The second approach is to look at absorption through follicular shunts. It is known that the penetration of NaCl through the haired abdominal skin of guinea pigs is 20% greater than that through the hairless skin behind the ears.[32] Feldmann and Maibach[33] found that, in humans, the penetration of labeled hydrocortisone, a polar compound, on the head (face and scalp) was considerably greater than on the forearm or trunk. This was mainly attributed to the high density of follicular shunts. Although the follicle openings comprise no more than 0.1 to 0.2% of the surface, the significance of the penetration of potent peptides via this route cannot be ignored.

The third approach is to investigate enhanced permeation through skin by using hydration enhancers such as dimethyl sulfoxide, Azone®, and surfactants, and by other physical means such as electrophoresis, streaming hot air flow, etc. Besides physical means, both skin hydration and enhancers for the permeation of low molecular drugs have been well documented in the literature. Some laboratories have started to investigate the possibility of insulin permeation through the skin, modulated by physical and/or mechanical means.

In short, transdermal administration of macromolecules is a desirable goal. Oral administration is not suitable in most cases, as drugs are destroyed in the digestive tract. Subdermal injections and implantation have inherent disadvantages, such as the discomfort of administration, the necessity for administration by trained personnel, and problems with patient compliance. However, there are technical difficulties with transdermal administration, due primarily to the poor diffusion characteristics of macromolecules which have not yet been overcome. At this moment, the outlook for transdermal delivery of macromolecules is pessimistic. However, with the rapid advances currently being made in this field, it may be possible at some future time to realistically consider this approach as an alternative and an improvement over the current methods of injection and implantation. Nevertheless, transdermal delivery will probably be restricted to the smaller peptides with low required doses.

REFERENCES

1. **Anon.,** Impacts of Applied Genetics: Micro-Organisms, Plants, and Animals, OTC Reports, Office of Technology Assessment, Congress of the United States, Washington, D.C., 1981.
2. **Goosen, T., O'Shea, G., Chou, S., and Sun, A.,** Slow release of insulin from biodegradable microbeads injected in diabetic rats, presented at the 10th Int. Symp. of Controlled Release of Bioactive Material, San Francisco, Calif., 1983.
3. **Sanders, L. M., Kent, J. S., McRae, G. I., Vickery, B. H., Tice, T. R., and Lewis, D. H.,** Controlled release of a luteinizing hormone-releasing hormone analogue from poly(d,l-lactide-co-glycolide) microspheres, *J. Pharm. Sci.,* 71, 1294, 1984.
4. **Longo, W. E., Iwata, H., Lindheimer, T. A., and Goldberg, E. P.,** Preparation of hydrophilic albumin microspheres using polymeric dispersing agents, *J. Pharm. Sci.,* 73, 1323, 1982.
5. **Schroeder, U. and Stahl, A.,** Crystallized dextran nanospheres with entrapped antigen and their use as adjuvants, *J. Immunol. Meth.,* 70, 127, 1984.
6. **Baker, R. W., Tuttle, M. E., and Helwing, R.,** Novel erodible polymers for the delivery of macromolecules, *Pharm. Technol.,* 8(2), 26, 1984.
7. **Rosen, H. B., Chang, J., Wnek, G. E., Linhardt, R. J., and Langer, R.,** Bioerodible polyanhydrides for controlled drug delivery, *Biomater. Med. Devices Artif. Organs,* 4, 131, 1983.
8. **Slavin, D.,** Production of antisera in rabbits using calcium alginate as an antigen depot, *Nature (London),* 165, 115, 1950.
9. **Goosen, M. F. A., Leung, Y. F., O'Shea, G. M., Chou, S., and Sun, A. M.,** Long-acting insulin: slow release of insulin from a biodegradable matrix implanted in diabetic rats, *Diabetes,* 32, 478, 1983.
10. **Leong, K. W., Cicuta, A., and Langer, R.,** Controlled release of bioactive agents from bioerodible polyanhydride microcapsules, presented at the 11th Int. Symp. on Controlled Release of Bioactive Materials, Ft. Lauderdale, Fla., 1984.
11. **Creque, H. M., Langer, R., and Folkman, J.,** One month sustained release of insulin from a polymer implant, *Diabetes,* 29, 37, 1980.
12. **Preis, I. and Langer, R.,** A single step immunization by sustained antigen release, *J. Immunol. Meth.,* 28, 193, 1979.
13. **Langer, R., Fefferman, M., Gryska, P. V., and Bergman, K.,** A simple method for studying chemotaxis using sustained release of attractants from inert polymers, *Can. J. Microbiol.,* 26, 274, 1980.
14. **Langer, R., Brem, H., Falterman, K., Klein, M,. and Folkman, J.,** Isolation of a cartilage factor that inhibits tumor neovascularization, *Science,* 193, 70, 1976.

15. **Ausprunk, D., Falterman, K., and Folkman, J.,** The sequence of events in the regression of corneal capillaries, *Lab. Invest.,* 38, 284, 1978.
16. **Hsieh, D. S. T., Langer, R., and Folkman, J.,** Magnetic modulation of release of macromolecules from polymers, *Proc. Natl. Acad. Sci. U.S.A.,* 78, 1863, 1981.
17. **Langer, R. and Folkman, J.,** Sustained release of macromolecules from polymers, in *Polymeric Delivery Systems,* Vol. 5, Kostelnik, R. J., Ed., Midland Macromolecular Monographs, Gordon and Breach Science, New York, 1978, 175.
18. **Hsieh, D. S. T., Chang, C. C., and Desai, D. S.,** Controlled release of macromolecules from silicone elastomer, *Pharm. Technol.,* 9(6), 39, 1985.
19. **Rhine, W. D., Hsieh, D. S. T., and Langer, R.,** Polymers for sustained macromolecule release: procedures to fabricate reproducible delivery systems and control release kinetics, *J. Pharm. Sci.,* 69, 265, 1980.
20. **Langer, R. and Folkman, J.,** Polymers for the sustained release of proteins and other macromolecules, *Nature (London),* 263, 797, 1976.
21. **Bawa, R. S.,** Controlled Release of Macromolecules from Ethylene-Vinyl Acetate Copolymer Matrices: Microstructure and Kinetic Analysis, Master's thesis, Massachusetts Institute of Technology, Cambridge, 1981.
22. **Hsieh, D. S. T., Rhine, W. D., and Langer, R.,** Zero-order controlled release polymer matrices for micro- and macro-molecules, *J. Pharm Sci.,* 72, 17, 1983.
23. **Rhine, W., Sukhatme, V., Hsieh, D. S. T., and Langer, R.,** A new approach to achieve zero-order release kinetics from polymer matrix drug delivery systems, in *Symposium on Controlled Release of Bioactive Materials,* Baker, R., Ed., Academic Press, New York, 1980, 177.
24. **Hsieh, D. S. T. and Langer, R.,** Zero-order drug delivery systems with magnetic control, in *Controlled Release Delivery Systems,* Mansdorf, S. Z. and Roseman, R. J., Eds., Marcel Dekker, New York, 1982, chap. 7, p. 121.
25. **Hsieh, D. S. T. and Langer, R.,** Methods of Making Prolonged Release Body, U.S. Patent 4,357,312.
26. **Hsieh, D. S. T. and Langer, R.,** Magnetic modulation of insulin release in diabetic rats, presented at the 9th Int. Symp. of Controlled Release of Bioactive Material, Ft. Lauderdale, Fla., 1982.
27. **Cohen, J., Siegel, R., and Langer, R.,** Sintering technique for the preparation of polymer matrices for the controlled release of macromolecules, *J. Pharm. Sci.,* 73, 1034, 1984.
28. **Colton, C. K., Satterfield, C. N., and Lai, C. J.,** Diffusion and partitioning of macromolecules within finely porous glass, *A.I.Ch.E. J.,* 21, 289, 1975.
29. **Kligman, A. M.,** A biological brief on percutaneous absorption, *Drug Dev. Ind. Pharm.,* 9, 521, 1983.
30. **Shaw, J.,** Development of transdermal therapeutic systems, *Drug Dev. Ind. Pharm.,* 9, 579, 1983.
31. **Barrow, G. M.,** *Physical Chemistry,* 3rd ed., McGraw-Hill, New York, 1973, p. 727.
32. **Wahlberg, J. E.,** Transepidermal or transfollicular absorption?, *Acta Derm. Venereol.,* 48, 336, 1968.
33. **Feldmann, R. J. and Maibach, H. I.,** Regional variations in percutaneous absorption of carbon-14 labelled cortisol in man, *J. Invest. Dermatol.,* 48, 181, 1967.

Index

INDEX

A

Abrasion of skin, 38
Absorbent pads, 125—126
Absorption
  continuous flow system, 66, 67
  dermal, 65, 67
  of nitroglycerin, 76, 131, 135, 136, 138
  percutaneous, see Percutaneous absorption
  of pesticides, 62
  skin dynamics of, 159
Activity/structure model, 54
Adhesion, 14—15, 125
  cell, 35
  in components of Nitro-Dur system, 125
  face, 14
  peripheral, 14
  pressure sensitive, 14, 125, 146
Adhesive diffusion-controlled systems, 88, 92
Adhesive layer, 86, 88
Adhesive rim, 89, 90
Advantages of transdermal delivery, 5—7, 102, 104
Age and skin condition, 74
Alginate, 172
Alkanoic acids, 53
Alkanol, 53
n-Alkanols, 53
n-Alkyl *p*-amino benzoates, 53
Aluminum foil package in Nitro-Dur system, 123
Alza-membrane system, 158
Amino acid precursors, 39
Anatomy of skin, 30—38
Angina pectoris treatment, see Nitroglycerin
Animal models, see also specific animals, 61—69,
    168
  dose evaluations in, 154
  in vitro, 62—65
  in vitro permeation kinetics in, 92—93
  in vivo, 65—68
  nitroglycerin dose evaluations in, 154
Annealing (heat-treatment), 22
Anomalous transport mechanisms, 24
Antimuscarinic drugs, see also specific types, 106
Apocrine gland, 32
Application site, 74—75
Application time, 76—78
Aqueous dispersion method, 179
Aqueous pore pathways, 56
Azone, 168, 192

B

Barriers of polymers, 122
Basal cells, 33—35
Basal lamina, 33
Basement membranes, 33
Benzoates, 53

Benzoic acid, 62, 63
Bicycle exerciser, 128
Binding, 56
  membrane, 58
Bioavailability, 72
  hair dye, 65
  in vivo, 94—95
  nitroglycerin, 73, 136, 137, 154—155
Biochemistry of skin, 39—40
Biphasic relationship for partitioning, 55
Blood concentrations
  of estradiol, 115
  of estrone, 115
  of nitroglycerin, 73, 126, 135, 136, 139
  of scopolamine, 106, 108
Blood supply to skin, 30—32
Branching
  degree of, 21
  effect of, 22

C

Callus tissue, 38
Cantharidine, 74
Carbohydrates, see also specific types, 39
Casting of solvents, 174—181
Catapres, 114
Categorization of polymeric systems, 8
Cell envelope, 36
Cells, see also specific types
  basal, 33—35
  diffusion, see Diffusion cells
  Franz, 52, 85, 91
  Langerhans', 37
  mast, 30
  Merkle, 37
  stratum corneum, 36
Cellular adhesion, 35
Cellulose triacetate, 161—168
Ceramides, 35
Changing membrane, 57
Chemical functionality of drug, 11
Chemical insult to skin, 38
Chemical treatment of membranes, 58
Chlorpheniramine, 15, 168
Choice of drugs, 11
Clearance, of nitroglycerin, 132
Clinical considerations, 71—78
Clinical dose, 76—77
Clinical improvements, 6—7
Clinical studies, 62
Clonidine, 105, 111—114
  multilaminate systems for, 106
  percutaneous absorption of, 88
  seven-day efficacy of, 112
  side effects of, 112
  technologies for, 106

Q

R